THE MEDICAL CARE OF TERMINALLY ILL PATIENTS

THE MEDICAL CARE OF TERMINALLY ILL PATIENTS

Second Edition

ROBERT E. ENCK, M.D.

Clinical Associate Professor
Hematology-Oncology Division, Department of Medicine
University of Pennsylvania School of Medicine
Philadelphia, Pennsylvania

Editor-in-Chief
American Journal of Hospice and Palliative Care

The Johns Hopkins University Press / Baltimore and London

Drug dosage: The author and publisher have exerted every effort to ensure that the selection and dosage of drugs discussed in this text accord with recommendations and practice at the time of publication. However, in view of ongoing research, changes in governmental regulations, and the constant flow of information relating to drug therapy and drug reactions, the reader is urged to check the package insert of each drug for any change in indications and dosage and for warnings and precautions. This is particularly important when the recommended agent is a new and/or infrequently used drug.

© 1994, 2002 The Johns Hopkins University Press
All rights reserved. First Edition 1994
Second edition 2002
Printed in the United States of America on acid-free paper
9 8 7 6 5 4 3 2 1

The Johns Hopkins University Press
2715 North Charles Street
Baltimore, Maryland 21218-4363
www.press.jhu.edu

Library of Congress Cataloging-in-Publication Data

Enck, Robert E.
    The medical care of terminally ill patients / Robert E. Enck.—
2nd ed.
        p.   cm.
    Includes bibliographical references and index.
    ISBN 0-8018-6765-7 (hardcover : alk. paper)—ISBN
    0-8018-6766-5 (pbk. : alk. paper)
    1.   Terminal care.
    [DNLM: 1. Palliative Care. 2. Terminal Care. WB 310 E56m
2002] I. Title.
    R726.8.E53 2002
    362.1'75—dc21
    00-013053

A catalog record for this book is available from the British Library.

How people die remains in the memories of those who live on.
Cicely Saunders, "Pain and Impending Death"

Contents

Preface to the Second Edition

Since the publication of *The Medical Care of Terminally Ill Patients* in 1994, significant social and scientific progress has been achieved, in caring for dying patients. Society continues to address the issue of physician-assisted suicide and euthanasia with the passage of the Oregon Death with Dignity Act and the conviction of Dr. Jack Kevorkian for murder. Although these events may be viewed as a mixed message regarding societal values on assisting death, at the very least the issues are now being publicly aired. Therefore, chapter 13 (Issues Concerning the Sustaining of Life) has been expanded. A review of the Oregon Death with Dignity Act experience reaches the somewhat surprising conclusion that the fear of intractable terminal pain is not a major factor in patients seeking physician-assisted suicide. Also, physician-assisted suicide and euthanasia, as practiced in the Netherlands, does not always result in a peaceful death.

Clearly, the medical community has responded to the public pressure for better education of physicians in terminal care. Numerous national initiatives, such as the American Medical Association's Education for Physicians on End-of-Life Care and the American College of Physicians–American Society of Internal Medicine End-of-Life Care Consensus Panel have been undertaken to educate physicians on good care for their dying patients. Palliative care textbooks and new journals proliferate, and a few academic institutions offer palliative care fellowships.

Likewise, incremental scientific gains in caring for the dying patient have occurred over the past five years. To reflect this, over 100 new references have been added to this second edition and, as in the previous edition, I have attempted to include those papers that are scientifically sound and clinically applicable to the terminal care setting. Unlike cancer treatment palliative care has seen few randomized clinical trials; in some cases, especially the adjuvant analgesics (chapter 8, Adjuvant Analgesic Drugs), the information is often anecdotal and extrapolated from one chronic disease to another. For example, gabapentin is a highly effective treatment for diabetic neuropathy and, based on this, is often used in neuropathy related to cancer. In other cases, such as the use and efficacy of herbs and vitamins by dying patients, virtually no data exist to substantiate their efficacy.

The growing appreciation of the poor prognosis associated with chronic congestive heart failure is reflected in the inclusion of this disease in chapter 1 (The Prognostication of Survival) and chapter 4 (Other Problems of Patients with Nonmalignant Diseases). The debate on the use of oxygen with the dying patient continues, as noted in chapter 2 (General Symptoms of Dying Patients). Although there are no new opioid drugs, the duration of administration has changed significantly to longer-acting preparations, and these, as well as the addition of the science on the use of oral transmucosal fentanyl for breakthrough pain are discussed in chapter 7 (Opioids). Newer information on the use of the bisphosphonates in managing metastatic bone pain is noted in chapter 10 (Bone Pain) and mention is made of complementary/alternative medicine in chapter 11 (Surgery and Other Nonpharmacologic Interventions to Manage Pain). As extensively reviewed in chapter 12 (The Final Moments), the controversy regarding terminal sedation appears to have subsided with a clearer understanding of its role in the terminally ill patient. In addition, there is a new list of abbreviations, information has been added to all the chapters, and the tables have been updated to include newer drugs and dosages.

As with the first edition, this book is the effort of a clinician writing for other clinicians. It is not a handbook, nor is it an all-encompassing textbook on the subject of terminal care. Rather, it reviews the results of clinical studies that are applicable to the management of the dying patient at the bedside. I hope that physicians and nurses will find this second edition useful in providing high-quality care for their patients as the end of life nears.

List of Abbreviations

ACE	angiotensin-converting enzyme
AIDS	acquired immunodeficiency syndrome
ALS	amyotrophic lateral sclerosis
AZT	azidothymidine (Zidovudine)
BUN	blood urea nitrogen
CAI	cardiovascular autonomic insufficiency
CAM	complementary/alternative medicine
CDC	Centers for Disease Control and Prevention
CMV	cytomegalovirus
CNS	central nervous system
CPR	cardiopulmonary resuscitation
CSF	cerebrospinal fluid
CSIM	continuous subcutaneous infusions of metoclopramide
CT	computed tomography
CTZ	chemoreceptor trigger zone
DAT	dementia of the Alzheimer type
DNR	do not resuscitate
ECOG	Eastern Cooperative Oncology Group
EMG	electromyogram
HDC	hypodermoclysis
HIV	human immunodeficiency virus
IM	intramuscular
IV	intravenous
JCAHO	Joint Commission on the Accreditation of Healthcare Organizations
KPS	Karnofsky Performance Status
MRI	magnetic resonance imaging
NBS	narcotic bowel syndrome
NG	nasogastric
NSAIDs	nonsteroidal anti-inflammatory drugs
OAF	osteoclast-activating factor
OTFC	oral transmucosal fentanyl citrate
PAS	physician-assisted suicide
PCA	patient-controlled analgesia

PSDA	Patient Self-Determination Act
PSYCOG	Psychosocial Collaborative Oncology Group
RMM	respiration with mandibular movement
SC	subcutaneous
SSRI	selective serotonin reuptake inhibitor
TCA	tricyclic antidepressant
TENS	transcutaneous electrical nerve stimulation
TNF	tumor necrosis factor
TTS	Transdermal Therapeutic System
WHO	World Health Organization

THE MEDICAL CARE OF TERMINALLY ILL PATIENTS

Chapter 1

The Prognostication of Survival

The problem of accurate prognosis has plagued hospice programs since the Medicare hospice benefit was enacted in 1982. The legislation provides Medicare coverage for a terminally ill patient whom a physician has certified to have a prognosis of six months or less to live. An inaccurate prognosis (i.e., the patient lives more than six months) results in a financial drain on the hospice. Shorter survival (in the range of days), which is common, deprives the patient and family of the true benefits of a hospice program. Indeed, as part of a national survey of nonparticipating hospices, the U.S. General Accounting Office (1989) indicated that one of the main concerns that led these hospices to choose not to participate in Medicare was the fact that the language required in hospice certification of terminal illnesses related to the certainty of the physician's prognosis of death. As a practical matter, many patients and families need to have some estimation of survival so the patient can get his or her affairs in order and allow appropriate time for good-byes.

In 1949, Karnofsky and Burchenal derived a numerical scale for quantifying a patient's functional status. This scale, now known as the Karnofsky Performance Status (KPS) scale, ranges from 0 to 100:

100 = normal; no complaints, no evidence of disease

90 = able to carry on normal activity; minor signs or symptoms of disease

80 = able to carry on normal activity with effort; some signs or symptoms of disease

70 = cares for self but is unable to carry on normal activity or do active work

60 = requires occasional assistance but is able to care for most of his or her needs

50 = requires considerable assistance and frequent medical care

40 = disabled; requires special care and assistance

30 = severely disabled; hospitalization is indicated, although death is not imminent

20 = very sick; hospitalization (active supportive treatment) is necessary

10 = moribund; fatal processes, progressing rapidly

0 = dead

In 1985, Evans and McCarthy reported the results of their prognostic studies in 42 terminally ill patients. The six members of a terminal care support team in a London health district reported both the upper and the lower estimates of prognosis, in days, for 42 patients during 149 visits, in addition to assessing the KPS score. The authors found that patients with KPS scores above 50 had a predicted survival of 24 days and those with scores of 50 or less survived between 3 and 70 days. Just over half of the actual survivals were within the estimated time, which tended to be overly optimistic. Evans and McCarthy concluded that KPS scores correlated more closely with actual survivals than did estimates provided by members of the terminal care support team.

Cancer

In 1980, Yates, Chalmer, and McKegney evaluated patients with advanced cancer using the KPS measurement. They studied 104 patients (42 women and 62 men, with an average age of 57 years). They collected a KPS score for each patient and then compared the score to the survival. It was clear that a low KPS score was strongly correlated with death within a relatively short time. Only 1 of the patients with a KPS score less than 50 survived longer than six months. However, a high KPS score was not predictive of long-term survival, because many of the patients with high initial scores died quickly. In addition, a patient's deterioration and subsequent death within a few months was predicted, to a limited degree, by a rapidly dropping KPS score.

In 1988 and 1989 Forster and Lynn reported the results of a study predicting survival for hospice inpatients. In their first paper (1988), two oncologists, a general internist, an oncology nurse, and a hospice social worker independently estimated the life span of 108 consecutive applicants for inpatient hospice care. The survival estimations were based on data in a 10-page multidisciplinary application packet. The actual median survival of the 108 patients was 3.5 ± 12.4 weeks. More than one-fourth of the patients died within 1 week of applying for hospice care, and only a small proportion lived beyond 12 weeks. The mean age of the sample was 66.2 years. Slightly more than half were women, and approximately the same proportion were white. The most common major symptoms and signs at the time of application were difficulty with ambulation, anemia, and pain. The survival predictions of the five member groups exceeded the actual survival by an average of 3.4 weeks. The authors speculated that this imprecision in expert estimation of life span poses substantial problems for hospice programs and policy makers.

In their second paper, Forster and Lynn (1989) extended their prior study. The authors collected data on 48 objective patient variables. They were particularly interested in defining objective variables that could distinguish between patients who were likely to die within either three or six months and those who were likely to live longer. These variables included primary neoplasm, hormone treatment, congestive heart failure, pain, disorientation, lack of funds, KPS score, respiratory disease, sodium level, admission to hospice, weakness, and sex. The KPS score and indication of weakness were the only two variables by logistic regression that contributed substantially to the probability of dying within three months. Using the six-month survival, the investigators found a correlation between women and those who had hormone treatments, indicating a high probability of living beyond six months.

Forster and Lynn (1989) suggested, based on this survival analysis and their research, that definable groups of applicants to hospice experienced different patterns of survival. They found a worse life expectancy among those with primary neoplasms involving the lung or colon, with disorientation, without congestive heart failure or hormone treatment, and with low sodium levels. Furthermore, the authors found that accurate prognostication of survival takes more precise knowledge than had been previously appreciated and that accuracy may be too limited for reliable forecasts for individual patients.

In 1988, Reuben, Mor, and Hiris published their research, as part of the National Hospice Study, on clinical symptoms and the length of survival of terminally ill cancer patients. The authors examined the correlation of 14 clinical symptoms with survival. The symptoms examined were nausea, dry mouth, anorexia, weight loss, difficulty swallowing, constipation, dizziness, fever, shortness of breath, diarrhea, hemorrhaging, bone pain, severe pain, and moderate or severe disorientation. Performance status was measured using the KPS scale. The sample frame was obtained from the National Hospice Study data set. Fifty-three percent of the study patients were women. The average age was 67 years. The KPS score was assessed by trained interviewers on the basis of their observation of the patients.

The authors reported that performance status was the most important clinical factor in estimating the survival time. Of the 14 clinical symptoms assessed, 5 had independent prognostic value: dyspnea, anorexia, dry mouth, difficulty swallowing, and weight loss. Based on these variables, the investigators developed four parametric accelerated time survival models to estimate the survival of patients with combinations of these symptoms and then validated the model on the entire data set. This model was not affected by a patient's age, sex, primary tumor site, or type. Reuben, Mor, and Hiris (1988) noted that their prediction rule seemed to be most valuable in estimating the length of survival for patients in the midlevel (KPS 30–40) and high-level (KPS $\geq$ 50) categories of performance status. In their study, 67 percent of the patients were at midlevel KPS. The predicted median survival time ranged from 36 days for patients with all five symptoms to 115 days for patients with none of the symptoms. Similarly, the predicted median survival time for the 17.5 percent of the patients in the highest KPS category was 54 days if all five symptoms were present and 172 days if none was present. For patients in the lowest KPS category (10–20), survival was poor regardless of the number of symptoms present: the predicted median survival time was 16 days if all five symptoms were present and 53 days if none was present. Hence, the authors concluded that the value of the model may be less for severely dysfunctional terminally ill patients.

Higginson, Wade, and McCarthy (1990) emphasized the importance of the Karnofsky index as a predictor of survival in terminal care. In their 487 patients, there was a clear trend of shorter survival with reducing mobility. When KPS ratings fell to 50 or below, 93 percent died within three months and 99 percent died within six months (table 1.1).

Recent research has focused on identifying interactions among KPS, symptom status, and quality-of-life measurements. Patients with lower KPS scores have more severe symptoms, a poorer quality of life, and more emotional distress. Symptom scales generally correlate well with the KPS rating. Symptoms may interact with the quality of life. For example, in cancer patients with moderate to severe pain, interference by pain has a

TABLE 1.1   Survival Time of Cancer Patients by Change in Karnofsky Performance Status (KPS)

KPS Score	Number of Patients	Survival (days) after Reaching Each KPS Score		
		Mean	Median	Range
80	5	48.6	52	20–69
70	43	48.1	39	0–175
60	96	43.3	29.5	0–344
50	167	30.9	17	0–491
40	204	20.3	11	0–379
30	169	14.8	6	0–372
20	127	11.9	6	0–365
10	80	10.8	2	0–365

Source: Higginson, Wade, and McCarthy (1990).

clear inverse relationship with the quality of life. These intertwined relationships challenge simplistic interpretations of how the quality of life or symptoms may predict survival (Chang 2000).

Several studies have addressed the issue of both physician and patient accuracy in predicting life expectancy. Weeks et al. (1998) prospectively studied 917 patients with advanced non–small cell lung cancer or colon cancer with liver metastases. They found that physicians were generally good at predicting a six-month survival, whereas 82 percent of patients overestimated their survival and 59 percent were extremely overly optimistic (Smith and Swisher 1998; Weeks et al. 1998). Christakis and Lamont (2000) asked 343 physicians to provide survival estimates for 468 terminally ill patients at the time of referral to five outpatient hospice programs in Chicago. The patients had a mean age of 69 years, and fewer than half (45%) were men. The diagnosis was cancer for 65 percent, acquired immunodeficiency syndrome (AIDS) for 12 percent, and other conditions for 23 percent. Median survival was 24 days. They found that only 20 percent of the prognoses were accurate. Most predictions (63%) were overly optimistic; only 17 percent were too pessimistic. Furthermore, they reported that the greater the experience of the physician, the better the prognostic accuracy, but a strong physician-patient relationship lowered this accuracy. Christakis and Lamont (2000) concluded that physicians are inaccurate in their prognosis for terminally ill patients and their error is systematically optimistic. An accompanying editorial (Parkes 2000) questioned the value of guessing short time survival by physicians in this study (Christakis and Lamont 2000) and encouraged the use of available prognostic indicators rather than intuition.

Dementia

The survival of patients with dementia of the Alzheimer type (DAT) is highly variable, often ranging from five to eight years. To study the clinical course of patients with DAT and to identify factors prognostic of survival, Walsh, Welch, and Larson (1990) prospectively evaluated and followed 200 outpatients with DAT at a university hospital. The mean age was 73.9 years at the onset of symptoms and 77.6 years at enrollment in the study. The median survival time from the onset of symptoms was 9.3 years, with a range of 1.8 to 16+ years, whereas the median survival time from enrollment in the study was 5.3 years, with a range of 0.2 to 7.2+ years. The severity of the dementia, as measured by the Mini-Mental State Examination (a 0 to 30–point scale, with 0 being the most cognitively impaired and 30 being the least impaired), correlated strongly with the survival time. The median survival time of patients with scores of 18 or less was three years shorter than that of patients with scores above 18. Factors found not to influence survival were the duration of symptoms, sex, depression, restlessness, comorbid conditions, vision problems, a reported decrease in appetite, the use of prescription drugs, and selected laboratory abnormalities (anemia, a low serum folate level, and an abnormal serum creatinine level).

A multivariate analysis of the age of onset of symptoms and of historical features showed that the combination of wandering and falling and the presence of behavioral problems at the time of evaluation appeared to affect survival adversely. The authors did not expect this finding, since patients with dementia are known to have a higher risk of falls and fractures than patients of the same age without dementia. These fractures often immobilize patients, which in turn leads to other potentially fatal complications, such as pulmonary embolus and aspiration pneumonia. The multivariate analysis suggested that behavioral problems were related to wandering and falling but were not as important in predicting survival. As noted by the authors, behavioral problems themselves and the management of them may be responsible for poor outcomes. For example, the use of sedative and hypnotic drugs to control agitation has been associated with falling and hip fracture (Ray et al. 1987).

Morrison and Siu (2000) investigated the issue of survival in end-stage dementia, be it DAT or vascular dementia, following an acute illness. Six-month mortality was 53 percent for patients with end-stage dementia and pneumonia, compared with 13 percent for cognitively intact patients. Six-month mortality was 55 percent for patients with end-stage dementia and hip fracture, compared with 12 percent for cognitively intact patients. Therefore, as reported by the authors, hip fracture and pneumonia are poor prognostic indicators for persons with advanced, end-stage dementia.

Motor Neuron Disease

O'Brien, Kelly, and Saunders (1992) retrospectively evaluated their experience with 124 patients with motor neuron disease cared for at St. Christopher's Hospice in London during a 12-year period. The age at the onset of the illness correlated significantly with survival, with younger patients living longer than older patients (table 1.2).

Acquired Immunodeficiency Syndrome (AIDS)

Because of the comparatively recent onset of the AIDS epidemic, few studies have systematically evaluated factors prognostic of the length of

TABLE 1.2   Survival Time Related to Patient's Age at the Onset of Motor Neuron Disease

Age of Onset (yr)	Number of Patients	Mean Survival (mo)
<40	3	77
40–49	15	77
50–59	30	48
60–69	43	35
70–7	27	28
>80	3	13
Total	121[a]	42

Source: O'Brien, Kelly, and Saunders (1992)
[a]Date of death unknown for three patients.

survival of the terminally ill patient with AIDS. To this end, Cole (1991) reviewed the medical literature to identify clinically significant indicators for survival (table 1.3). Clearly, there is wide variation in survival with complicating diseases such as Kaposi sarcoma and non-Hodgkin lymphoma, which reflects the degree of underlying impairment of the patient's immune system. For example, the prognosis for Kaposi sarcoma occurring in patients with no concurrent opportunistic infection and little immune dysfunction is more favorable (median survival of 31 months) than that of the same tumor seen in patients with advanced AIDS (median survival of 7 months).

   Mocroft et al. (1997) studied 2,625 patients with AIDS in two large London hospitals between 1982 and July 1995. They found that the median survival (20 months) was longer than previous estimates and that the CD4 count at diagnosis significantly decreased over time.

Central Nervous System Anoxia

   Global central nervous system anoxia, often following cardiopulmonary arrest, may lead to a chronic vegetative state, with hopelessness for the family and an array of distressing symptoms for the patient. Longstreth et al. (1983) retrospectively studied the neurologic sequelae of out-of-hospital cardiac arrest, looking at 459 consecutive patients admitted to a teaching hospital over ten years. One hundred and eighty patients (39%) never awakened and 279 (61%) awakened, 188 without and 91 with persistent neurologic deficits. Patients who never awoke had a median survival of 3.5 days. The longer a comatose patient survived, the smaller the chance of ever awakening or of awakening without deficits. In another study, Levy et al. (1985) investigated the outcome of coma

TABLE 1.3   The Prognostic Indicators of Survival Time in Patients with AIDS

Coexisting Condition	Survival (mo)
Opportunistic infection	
Pneumocystis carinii pneumonia	24[a]
Mycobacterium avium intracellulare	7[b]
Tumor	
Kaposi sarcoma	7–31
Non-Hodgkin lymphoma	6.8–24
Other complication	
AIDS-related dementia	1.8
Neurologic abnormalities	2.1
Constant diarrhea	3.2
Hypoxia (p02 $\leq$ 50 mm Hg)	1.0
Low serum albumin (<20 grams/L)	0.7
Peripheral blood pancytopenia[c]	2.5

Source: Cole (1991).

[a]Mean.

[b]Median.

[c]lymphocytes <1.5 × 10/L, hemocrit 30%, white blood cells <2.5 × 10 9/L and platelets <140 × 10 9/L.

after cardiac arrest in 210 patients and were able to develop simple prognostication rules for this clinical situation. Patients who, with initial examination or after 24 hours, had pupillary light reflexes, the development of spontaneous eye movements, and withdrawal response to pain experienced favorable outcomes.

Central nervous system anoxia may occur as a result of traumatic brain injury, the most common cause of death and disability in young individuals (Ghajar 2000). A poor prognosis is associated with coma and with inability of the patient to open his or her eyes or to follow commands within 24 hours of the injury. In addition, there is an increased risk of a poor outcome with advancing age, especially over the age of 60 years. Hypotension on admission to a hospital is associated with a doubling of the mortality risk. Finally, fixed and dilated (>4mm) pupils are associated with a 90 percent mortality.

Advanced Pulmonary Disease

Some 70 to 80 percent of persons with advanced pulmonary disease die within five years (Bergner et al. 1988). As noted by Kinzel (1991), prognostication is even more difficult for persons with advanced lung disease than for persons with cancer. Indeed, one study showed estimates varying from one month to five years in similar patients. Fox et al. (1999) highlighted this finding in their study of seriously ill hospitalized patients with advanced chronic obstructive pulmonary disease, congestive heart failure, and end-stage liver disease. They found that no clinical predictors were effective in identifying patients with a survival of six months or less. Nonetheless, several factors have been consistently associated with a limited survival for patients with advanced pulmonary disease (Schonwetter and Jani 2000):

- decreased FEV1,
- the presence of cor pulmonale,
- repeated episodes of respiratory failure,
- poor nutritional status.

Other factors that may be related to life expectancy in these patients include poor functional status, hypoxemia, psychological distress, polycythemia, resting tachycardia, decreased vital capacity, and continued smoking.

Heart Disease

As noted by Fox et al. (1999), there are no reliable clinical indicators to prognosticate six months or less survival for persons with congestive heart failure. Generally, persons dying with cancer have a long period of functional stability; a rapid decline in functional status occurs some one to three weeks before death (Morris et al. 1986). By comparison, persons with congestive heart failure often experience a slow and lengthy decline in daily functions interrupted by periodic bouts of severe symptoms and disability. Most deaths due to congestive heart failure occur suddenly and often unpredictably from arrhythmia (Lynn 1997).

Summary

No matter what the disease, the prognostication of survival is an inexact science widely influenced by individual patient variation. Studies of survival estimates made by physicians are inconclusive, ranging from accurate to overly optimistic predictions. On the other hand, patients tend to overestimate their actual survival.

For patients with advanced cancer, a low KPS score usually reflects a life span of a few weeks to days. In the more ambulatory and mobile patients (i.e., those with a middle to high KPS score), accurate prognostication of survival is more difficult. Therefore, like pain assessment, on-going measurement of KPS scores is an important clinical tool to monitor prognosis, especially as the scores decline.

The survival of patients with dementia of the Alzheimer type is highly variable. The severity of the dementia correlates strongly with survival: patients with milder dementia live significantly longer than do those more severely affected. Also, the presence of behavioral problems, the combination of wandering and falling at the time of the initial evaluation, and hospitalization for hip fracture or pneumonia adversely influence survival.

For patients with motor neuron disease, the length of life correlates inversely with the age of onset, with younger patients living longer than older patients.

Survival of persons with AIDS is variable, but appears to relate to the degree of impairment of the immune system. Patients with marked immune dysfunction as evidenced by the presence of opportunistic infection and malignancy survive for months.

Recovery from central nervous system anoxia following cardiopulmonary arrest directly relates to the patient's initial or 24-hour neurologic status. Improvement in this status denotes a favorable outcome, whereas persisting coma suggests a short survival.

Finally, the prognostication of survival for persons with advanced pulmonary disease or congestive heart failure is extremely difficult, and survival may range from months to years.

PART I

The Management of Symptoms Common among Dying Patients

Chapter 2

General Symptoms of Dying Patients

PAIN

Of all the symptoms encountered in dying patients, pain is the most common. It is discussed extensively in part II.

GASTROINTESTINAL SYMPTOMS

Nausea and Vomiting

Patients with advanced disease frequently experience nausea and vomiting. If unabated, these symptoms lead to serious nutritional problems, dehydration, and overall physical discomfort. In patients with cancer, these symptoms are generally associated with the use of chemotherapy. Much research effort has been devoted to developing various regimens of antiemetic drugs to control this distressing but time-limited side effect.

What has not been well studied or even well appreciated is the incidence of non-chemotherapy-induced nausea and vomiting in patients dying from advanced cancer. Reuben and Mor (1986b) shed some light on this subject as part of the National Hospice Study, which prospectively followed cancer patients over their last weeks of life. The authors found that 62 percent of terminally ill cancer patients experienced nausea and vomiting at some point in the last two months of life. Nausea and vomiting were reported more often in the following groups: patients with stomach or breast cancer as the primary type, women (even after excluding those with breast cancer), and patients younger than age 65. Approximately 25 percent of the patients in this study were receiving chemotherapy, and no association was observed between the chemotherapy and the reporting of nausea and vomiting at any time during the last six weeks of life. This finding suggests that the pathogenesis of chemotherapy-induced nausea and vomiting may differ from that due to terminal cancer itself. Of the

subset of nauseated patients, only 32 percent received an antiemetic prescription for a phenothiazine or an antihistamine. Physicians were more
hesitant to prescribe antiemetic drugs for elderly patients and those with
impaired levels of awareness. The results of this study imply that better
physician awareness may promote earlier therapeutic intervention to
help alleviate these symptoms in patients with terminal cancer.

Etiologies

With the recognition and early identification of the problem of nausea and vomiting, attention can be directed toward identifying the various etiologies of the symptoms and then treating the symptoms. Frequently, the cause of nausea and vomiting in the cancer patient is
multifactorial (table 2.1).

TABLE 2.1   Common Etiologies of Nausea and Vomiting in Patients with Advanced
Disease

Fluid and electrolyte disturbances
   Hypercalcemia
   Volume depletion
   Water intoxication (syndrome of inappropriate ADH[a] secretion)
   Adrenocortical insufficiency
Gastrointestinal
   Mouth: infections (*candida albicans,* herpes simplex) and ulceration
   Taste: postchemotherapy and tumor effect
   Esophagus: fungal infections, obstruction, and postradiation therapy inflammation
   Gastric: irritation and stasis
   Obstruction of the small bowel
   Constipation
Pancreatic carcinoma—gastric stasis
Hepatic metastases
Peritonitis
Central nervous system metastases
   Brain
   Meninges
Renal failure with uremia
Local infections and septicemia
Tumor toxins
Drugs
   Opioid analgesics
   Other medications (e.g., digoxin, nonsteroidal anti-inflammatories)
Radiation therapy, especially treatment of the gastrointestinal tract
Syndrome of cardiovascular autonomic insufficiency
Behavioral/psychogenic problems

Sources: Frytak and Moertel (1981); Bruera et al. (1986a); Allan (1988).
[a]ADH, antidiuretic hormone.

Frytak and Moertel (1981) emphasized the diagnostic subtleties of several of these causative factors, such as fluid and electrolyte disturbances, hypercalcemia, adrenocortical insufficiency, and meningeal metastases. This etiologic morass is often compounded by the addition of both opioid and nonopioid analgesic drugs to control pain. Indeed, in the World Health Organization's two-year experience with the analgesic ladder for cancer pain, nausea and vomiting were present in 22 percent of the days during the three-step treatment (Ventafridda et al. 1987). Furthermore, it seems that the incidence of nausea and vomiting is markedly increased in ambulatory patients treated with opioid analgesics.

A possible etiology for nausea and vomiting may be the presence of the syndrome of cardiovascular autonomic insufficiency (CAI). The clinical spectrum of CAI includes cardiovascular manifestations (postural hypotension, syncope, fixed heart rate) and gastrointestinal symptoms (nausea, anorexia, constipation, diarrhea). This syndrome is usually found in neurologic disorders, chronic renal disease, and diabetes mellitus. However, Bruera et al. (1986b) studied a group of breast cancer patients for the presence of CAI and identified this as a frequent feature in advanced cancer. The nausea, mostly chronic in CAI, was attributed to gastroparesis or a significantly prolonged gastric emptying time.

MANAGEMENT

Ideally, the management of nausea and vomiting is dependent on identifying and correcting the underlying etiologies (e.g., the use of corticosteroids for adrenocortical insufficiency, antibiotics for infection, and the like). In reality, the major problem is that in many cases the etiologies are multifactorial and often uncorrectable, as in the case of a patient with advanced metastatic liver disease on opioid analgesics. Therefore, the next step is the use of antiemetic drug therapy to control the symptoms.

The mechanism for controlling vomiting consists of two separate areas in the brain: the emetic center and the chemoreceptor trigger zone (CTZ) (Seigel and Longo 1981). The emetic center is the final common pathway that mediates all vomiting. In addition to input from the CTZ to the emetic center, the vestibular apparatus, the periphery (pharynx and gastrointestinal tract), and the cerebral cortex can induce emesis through the emetic center (fig. 2.1). Based on the extensive experience with the management of chemotherapy-induced nausea and vomiting, we can categorize antiemetic drugs as shown in table 2.2 (Seigel and Longo 1981; Dodds 1985).

Pharmacologic Treatment. The pharmacologic treatment of patients with nausea and vomiting is similar in many respects to that of patients

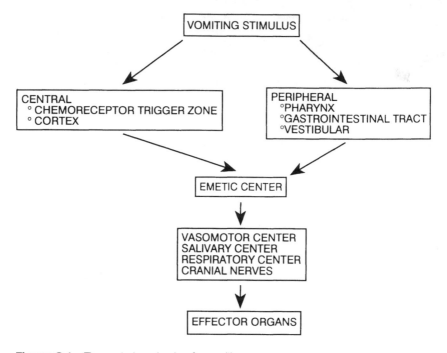

Figure 2.1.   The control mechanism for vomiting

with chronic pain, especially in regard to round-the-clock dosing and identifying patterns of the symptoms. It is difficult to generalize broadly based principles for the management of these patients because of the complexity of the problem. However, the following guidelines may be useful:

- The phenothiazines, such as prochlorperazine and thiethylperazine, are widely used antiemetic drugs, and the clinician should give them initial consideration. Many of the phenothiazines as well as the antihistamines are available in liquid as well as suppository form.
- If nausea and vomiting are related to opioid analgesics such as morphine, antiemetic drugs can be added, similar to the use of prochlorperzine with the Brompton mixture (Melzack, Mount, and Gordon 1979). However, the clinician should exercise care, since the antiemetic drugs may potentiate the side effects of the opioid analgesics.
- If the clinician suspects the syndrome of CAI and gastroparesis, treatment with metoclopramide is appropriate, since this drug accelerates gastric emptying (Kris et al. 1985).

TABLE 2.2   Antiemetic Drugs for the Management of Nausea and Vomiting

Pharmacologic Classification	Example	Proposed Site(s) of Action	Usual Dose
Antihistamines	Diphenhydramine	? Emetic center/ cortex/vestibular	50–100 mg PO, IM, IV every 6–8h
Anticholinergic medications	Scopolamine	? Emetic center/ vestibular	Transdermal patch (0.5 mg) every 3 days
Dopamine antagonists			
Phenothiazines	Prochlorperazine	CTZ	5–20 mg PO or IM every 4–6h
Butyrophenones	Haloperidol	CTZ	0.5–2 mg every 4–12h
Benzamides	Metoclopramide	Periphery/CTZ	10–15 mg PO every 6h
Cannabinoids	Dronabinol (delta-9-tetrahydrocannabinol)	Cortex	2.5–10 mg PO every day
Corticosteroids	Dexamethasone	?	10–20 mg IV × 1
Benzodiazepines	Lorazepam	Cortex	1–2 mg PO, IV every 6–8h
5-HT$_3$ antagonist	Ondansetron	Peripheral	4–8 mg PO or IV every 8–12h
Somatostatin	Octreotide	Peripheral	150–300 μg SC every 12h or 300–600 μg/24h continuous SC infusion

Sources: Data from Seigel and Longo (1981); Dodds (1985); Marin, Ilanez, and Arribas (1990); Abrahm (2000).
Note: CTZ, chemoreceptor trigger zone; IM, intramuscular; IV, intravenous; 5-HT, serotonin receptor; PO, oral; SC, subcutaneous

- Patients with a history of motion sickness appear to be more susceptible to nausea and vomiting (Dodds 1985) and therefore may benefit from drug therapy that acts at the vestibular center, such as the antihistamines or the anticholinergics.
- Nausea and vomiting due to malignant intestinal obstruction are difficult to treat, but the use of continuous-infusion antiemetic drugs seems to offer some relief (Baines, Oliver, and Carter 1985). If this fails and the total volume of vomitus is large, octreotide is often used. It is antisecretory and proabsorbtive, and reduces forward peristalsis. It can also be combined with other drugs for subcutaneous infusion (Baines 1997).
- For recalcitrant, intractable cases, a trial of continuous-infusion metoclopramide may be worthwhile in view of Warrington et al.'s (1986) experience in controlling chemotherapy-induced nausea and vomiting with this technique. Also, the combination of dexamethasone, metoclopramide, and hydroxyzine or diphenhydramine may be effective (Abrahm 2000).

Pharmacologic intervention infrequently causes adverse reactions, the most common being extrapyramidal. Holmes, Adams, and Fernandez (1987) reported the unusual occurrence of respiratory dyskinesia and akathisia after the use of the butyrophenone droperidol as an antiemetic. Both respiratory dyskinesia and akathisia are acute extrapyramidal reactions due to droperidol. Respiratory dyskinesia is characterized by difficulty breathing and a gasping sensation that is frequently misdiagnosed as agitation or anxiety. Both of these extrapyramidal reactions respond promptly to anticholinergic drugs. The 5-HT_3 antagonists, such as ondansetron, have no associated extrapyramidal reactions but can cause constipation and dose-related headache.

Nonpharmacologic Treatment. The nonpharmacologic management of nausea and vomiting is even less well delineated, and again the bulk of experience is extrapolated from the chemotherapy literature. Behavioral modification such as systemic desensitization is not practical in view of the length of time necessary to complete the procedure. To minimize or control, to some degree, the nausea and vomiting, the clinician may instruct the patient and the family to do the following (Hogan 1986):

- Use interventions that have helped relieve nausea and vomiting during pregnancy, illness, or times of stress. Often a particular food or beverage associated with a past positive experience may effectively relieve the nausea.
- Eat cold foods or foods served at room temperature, such as sandwiches, cottage cheese, cereals, and desserts. These foods are usually tolerated better than warm or hot foods, since the odors of hot foods often aggravate the feeling of nausea.
- Use a clear liquid diet to reduce nausea. Liquids such as apple juice, cranberry juice, lemonade, fruit ades, broth, ginger ale, tea, or cola are usually well tolerated. They should be sipped slowly. Bland foods such as popsicles, gelatin, mashed potatoes, applesauce, sherbet, crackers, toast, and cottage cheese are also well tolerated.
- Experiment with sour foods, such as lemons, sour pickles, hard sour candy, or lemon sherbet. The mouth can be rinsed with a mixture of lemon juice and water if stomatitis is not present.
- Avoid sweet, fatty, highly salted, and spicy foods as well as foods with strong odors.
- Minimize stimuli such as sights, sounds, or smells that can initiate nausea (e.g., unpleasant odors, strong perfume, other persons who are nauseated or vomiting, or the smell of food being cooked).
- Have the patient obtain fresh air by sitting near an open window or outside.

- Provide distraction. Enjoyable music, a favorite television program, electronic games, talking with others, and reading are examples of effective distractions. Describing a favorite place, one's home, or a person who is significant can also provide distraction.
- Use techniques such as relaxation response, with or without positive visual imagery.

Anorexia and Cachexia

Anorexia, or diminished appetite, is a common finding in patients with advanced cancer. One study (Curtis, Krech, and Walsh 1991) identified anorexia in 55 percent of 100 oncology patients. The symptom of anorexia itself inevitably leads to weight loss, which in turn accelerates a loss of tissue mass, resulting in cachexia. This vicious cycle of anorexia-weight loss-cachexia, often referred to as the anorexia-cachexia syndrome, is difficult to break and becomes self-perpetuating, resulting in the common clinical picture of the emaciated, malnourished, dying patient.

Much scientific interest and enthusiasm has been generated regarding this problem. In a large multicenter study, the Eastern Cooperative Oncology Group (ECOG) studied the prognostic effect of weight loss before chemotherapy in 3,047 patients enrolled in 12 chemotherapy protocols (DeWys et al. 1980). The frequency of weight loss ranged from 31 percent for favorable non-Hodgkin lymphoma to 87 percent for gastric carcinoma. The median survival was significantly shorter in nine protocols for patients with weight loss compared to patients with no weight loss. Chemotherapy response rates were lower in patients with weight loss, but only in breast cancer patients was this difference significant. In short, the ECOG study clearly delineated the importance of weight loss as a prognostic factor across many institutions.

ETIOLOGIES

As a result of the ECOG research endeavor, a better understanding of the pathophysiology of the anorexia-cachexia syndrome has evolved. It is apparent that the etiologies of this syndrome are multiple and frequently overlapping. Three major causative components have been identified: systemic effects of cancer, local effects of cancer, and treatment-related complications (Rivlin, Shils, and Sherlock 1983).

The systemic effect of cancer is a frequent occurrence in clinical practice. This remote effect of tumor is thought to be a paraneoplastic syndrome, in the sense that a tumor-associated substance is the causative agent(s). Elements of the anorexia-cachexia syndrome include weight loss, weakness, asthenia, anemia, and abnormalities of protein, lipid, and carbohydrate metabolism. The patient with this syndrome develops a negative energy balance in which the food intake is inappropriately less than the energy output, resulting in the net effect of loss of body weight (Langstein and Norton 1991). It has been suggested that tumor necrosis factor (TNF) is one such substance contributing to the development of cancer-associated cachexia. Animal studies provided strong circumstantial evidence linking TNF with this problem. However, conflicting results have been reported regarding the presence of TNF in the serum of randomly selected cancer patients. Socher et al. (1988) assayed TNF levels in serum from 19 patients who had weight losses ranging from 8 to 40 percent of their preillness weight. This weight loss was not attributable to anticancer therapy, gastrointestinal disorder, or other medical problems. The investigators detected no TNF in serum samples from the 19 patients studied. Despite copious research, no specific agent has been conclusively identified. It is most likely that multiple cytokines, such as TNF, interleukin-1, interleukin-6, and gamma-interferon, will be implicated in an interrelated fashion (Langstein and Norton 1991).

The local effects of cancer are generally mechanical or obstructive, depending on the tumor site. For example, patients with head and neck cancer may have difficulty swallowing, and those with gastrointestinal cancers may experience dysphagia, early satiety, obstruction, and malabsorption.

Finally, problems arising from the treatment of cancer may contribute to the anorexia-cachexia syndrome. Radiation therapy, especially to the oropharyngeal area, to the lower neck and mediastinum, and to the abdomen and pelvis, may cause significant nutritional problems, which are generally self-limited in time. Surgical procedures such as intestinal resection or bypass procedures of the small and large bowel cause more longstanding and chronic nutritional problems. Chemotherapy, like radiation therapy, may cause short periods of nutritional impairment usually related to drug-induced nausea and vomiting. Uncontrolled pain as well as the use of opioids to control pain may worsen the anorexia-cachexia syndrome.

By the time a patient is terminally ill, the contribution of cancer therapy to the anorexia-cachexia syndrome is less significant than either the systemic or the local effects of cancer. What is often perceived at this point as related to treatment is in reality the clinical consequences of unopposed tumor growth.

MANAGEMENT

Treatment options of the anorexia-cachexia syndrome and related nutritional problems in dying patients are slowly improving. Certainly the use of intensive parenteral or enteral hyperalimentation has little value for the dying patient. The American College of Physicians (1989) concluded that the routine use of parenteral nutrition for patients undergoing chemotherapy should be strongly discouraged, and, in deciding to use such therapy for individual patients whose malnutrition is judged to be life threatening, physicians should take into account the possibility of increased risk.

Until recently, there were few publications in the medical literature regarding drug therapy for the anorexia-cachexia syndrome. What was published was mostly anecdotal. Several reports have suggested possible roles for corticosteroids, megestrol acetate, and dronabinol.

Corticosteroids. Corticosteroids have been used widely for years to alleviate the symptoms of cachexia and weakness in cancer patients, but without sound, scientific backing. For example, Schell (1972) strongly advocated the widespread use of corticosteroids by patients dying with advanced cancer because it not only increased appetite and a sense of well-being but also reduced the inflammatory response and opioid requirements. In 1982, Derogatis and MacDonald, reporting for an American Cancer Society workshop, suggested the performance of prospective clinical trials on the use of corticosteroids by dying patients. In addition, they rightly pointed out that corticosteroids may cause symptoms of weakness and delirium, which are also commonly seen in patients with advanced cancer.

One of the earliest controlled and randomized studies of the use of corticosteroids for patients with advanced cancer was reported in 1974 by Moertel et al. from the Mayo Clinic. They studied 116 patients with far-advanced gastrointestinal cancer as part of a controlled, double-blind study comparing oral dexamethasone, 0.75 mg and 1.5 mg four times daily, to placebo. Two weeks after the start of treatment, more than half of the patients (57%) treated with dexamethasone reported an improvement in appetite and more than one-fourth (26%) reported improved strength. However, this improvement may have been in large measure a placebo effect, since a substantial proportion of patients treated with the inactive placebo compound also reported improvement. By the fourth week, much of the initial improvement of symptoms in the placebo-treated patients had lessened and the dexamethasone-treated patients showed a substantial and significant advantage. According to the authors, this improvement of symptoms was largely the result of dexamethasone-induced euphoria, as only three dexamethasone-treated patients had gained weight and only two noted an improvement in their performance status. Finally, the investigators felt that corticosteroid therapy did produce some improvement of symptoms in preterminal cancer patients with little discernible price in terms of side effects.

In 1984, Willox et al. studied 61 patients complaining of poor appetite or weight loss. The study was a double-blind, cross-over trial involving oral prednisolone, 5 mg three times daily for two weeks and then for a third week when the dosage was reduced, versus placebo. Forty-one of the 61 patients were evaluable: 16 men and 25 women, with an age range of 27 to 80 (mean 60) years. Prednisolone was found to be significantly better than placebo in improving appetite during the three weeks of the study. This improvement was also seen when patients who had been taking placebo crossed over to receive prednisolone. There was a major placebo effect in half the patients regarding improvement in appetite, which the authors interpreted as confirming a psychological basis for anorexia in some patients. Weight gain did not occur in either group of patients. When taking prednisolone, patients showed a trend toward increased food intake and a significant increase in well-being. Finally, none of the patients reported any side effects.

In a more complex study, Bruera et al. (1985) explored the efficacy of oral methylprednisolone in a prospective, randomized trial in terminally ill cancer patients. A 14-day, double-blind, cross-over protocol was used to test methylprednisolone, 16 mg twice daily, against placebo. Forty patients were entered on the study, and 31 were evaluable (12 men and 19 women, with a mean age of 51 years). The authors found that appetite increased in 24 patients (77%). However, they observed no change of nutritional status and no serious toxicity during the study. They concluded that a short course (two weeks) of methylprednisolone increased the comfort of severely symptomatic patients with advanced cancer.

Della Cuna, Pellegrini, and Piazzi (1989) reported the effectiveness of an eight-week course of 125 mg of intravenous methylprednisolone per day in improving the quality of life of patients with preterminal cancer. This was a double-blind, placebo-controlled, multicenter study. Quality of life was assessed by several instruments. A total of 403 patients were enrolled in the study, with 207 being treated with methylprednisolone and 196 receiving placebo. Overall, methylprednisolone was significantly more effective than placebo in improving the quality of life, as judged by the changes from baseline in the quality-of-life scales. Although an improvement in appetite was reported more frequently in the methylprednisolone group, there was no significant difference between this treatment and placebo in regard to changes in body weight.

In a second and related study, Popiela, Lucchi, and Giongo (1989) treated 173 terminally ill female cancer patients with either methylprednisolone or placebo. The methylprednisolone, at a dosage of 125 mg/day, was administered intravenously for eight consecutive weeks. Data were collected relative to the quality of life and other parameters. Eighty-five and 88 patients were randomized to treatment with methylprednisolone and placebo, respectively. As in the prior study, appetite showed consistent, often statistically significant, improvement across time in the methylprednisolone patients compared to the placebo group. However, this study did not monitor changes in weight.

Megestrol Acetate. Megestrol acetate is an oral progestational agent generally used in a dosage of 160 mg/day for diseases such as metastatic breast, endometrial, and renal cancer. It is well tolerated by patients except for occasional weight gain. Preliminary information suggested that megestrol acetate stimulates appetite and leads to nonfluid weight gain in some patients with metastatic breast and other cancers, as well as in those with acquired immunodeficiency syndrome (AIDS).

As part of a phase I and II trial studying the use of megestrol acetate in high dose as a treatment for breast cancer, Tchekmedyian et al. (1987) noted the presence of improved appetite and marked weight gain in these patients. The authors subsequently analyzed the pattern of weight change and the relationships of different variables to this weight change in those 28 patients with metastatic breast cancer treated with oral megestrol acetate (480 to 1,600 mg daily). Marked weight gain, ranging from 2 to 44 pounds, was noted, and enhanced appetite was found in 96 percent of the patients. Weight gain occurred regardless of the pretreatment weight, extent of metastases, or response to therapy. Although these results were preliminary, the authors suggested a possible role for megestrol acetate in reversing anorexia and weight loss, thus improving the quality of life of patients with cachexia.

Loprinzi et al. (1990) studied 133 patients with advanced, incurable cancer treated with either megestrol acetate or placebo. Entry into this randomized, double-blind, placebo-controlled trial required that each patient must have lost at least 5 pounds in the preceding two months or less and/or have had an estimated daily calorie intake of less than 20 Kcal/kg. Also, the attending physician must have determined that weight gain would have been beneficial to the patient. This multicenter, cooperative study (the North Central Cancer Treatment Group and the Mayo Clinic) included adult patients with advanced cancer except those with breast or endometrial sites. Before randomization, patients were stratified by primary site of disease, severity of weight loss, sex, and treatment with concurrent chemotherapy. Patients randomized to the megestrol acetate arm received 800 mg daily in three divided doses. The investigators collected extensive information, including a patient questionnaire.

In the group treated with megestrol acetate, 11 of 67 (16%) gained at least 15 pounds, with 3 patients gaining more than 30 pounds. Only one (2%) of the 66 patients treated with placebo gained this much. This difference was highly significant statistically. Of the patients in the megestrol acetate group, 16 percent gained 10 percent or more of their baseline weight, whereas no patients receiving placebo gained as much. There were no indications that the weight gain in these patients was related to the accumulation of excess fluid, such as ascites, edema, or pleural effusions. In those patients receiving concurrent chemotherapy, tumor regressions were not responsible for most of the weight gain seen in the study.

The investigators assessed the possibility of interaction between study treatment and each of the following factors: sex, age, primary tumor site, entry weight loss, performance status, and concurrent chemotherapy. They discovered no statistically significant interactions.

Toxicities were closely monitored. Patients in the megestrol acetate group experienced less nausea and emesis than did patients in the placebo group. Edema occurred more often in patients randomized to megestrol acetate (29% versus 13%), but clinically it was usually minimal and promptly responded to treatment with mild diuretics. Other possible side effects from megestrol acetate, such as impotence, irregular menses, and hypertension, were infrequent. No thrombotic events were noted in the patients receiving megestrol acetate. On the questionnaire, patients in the megestrol acetate group reported significantly better results for all questions related to appetite than did those assigned the placebo.

The authors thought that this study convincingly confirms that megestrol acetate can improve the appetite of patients with anorexia and cachexia associated with cancer and led to substantial weight gain in some of these patients. Surprisingly, the study found an impressive and statistically significant reduction in nausea (38% versus 13%) and vomiting (25% versus 8%) in patients assigned to receive megestrol acetate. The authors speculated that megestrol acetate stimulates appetite, which in turn reduces the nausea and vomiting attributable to advanced malignant disease.

The optimal dosage of megestrol acetate to stimulate appetite in patients with advanced cancer seems to be 800 mg/day. Prior studies in women with breast cancer suggest that there is a dose-response effect, and current research is ongoing in this area. Loprinzi et al. (1990) noted that treatment with 800 mg/day of megestrol acetate costs approximately $15 to $20 per day. An unanswered question is whether reversal of the anorexia and cachexia associated with advanced cancer will ultimately improve patient survival. In an updated study, Loprinzi et al. (1992) reported the results of a second North Central Cancer Treatment Group and Mayo Clinic trial, comparing three doses of megestrol acetate in patients with advanced cancer. A total of 343 eligible patients who had lost at least 5 pounds in the previous two months or had a caloric intake of less than 20 Kcal/kg were randomized to receive megestrol acetate dosages of 160 mg/day (88 patients), 480 mg/day (86 patients), or 1,280 mg/day (84 patients). Treatment groups were well balanced for prognostic factors. A positive dose-response effect on the patients' appetite and food intake was observed as the dosage of megestrol acetate increased from 160 mg/day to 800 mg/day. The data did not provide any support for dosages greater than 800 mg/day.

Addressing the issue of whether megestrol acetate offers an advantage over corticosteroids, Loprinzi et al. (1999) reported the results of a randomized trial comparing megestrol acetate and the corticosteroids dexamethasone and fluoxymesterone. They chose the anabolic steroid fluoxymesterone because it had been shown to increase muscle mass. Cancer patients with anorexia and cachexia were randomized to receive either dexamethasone 0.75 mg qid, megestrol acetate 800 mg orally every day, or fluoxymesterone 10 mg orally bid. In the 475 evaluable patients, they found that fluoxymesterone resulted in significantly less appetite enhancement and its toxicity profile was not better than that of the other two drugs studied. Megestrol acetate and dexamethasone caused the same degree of appetite stimulation and nonfluid weight status. Dexamethasone was noted to have more corticosteroid-type toxicity and/or patient refusal than megestrol acetate. On the other hand, megestrol acetate had a higher rate of deep vein thrombosis than did dexamethasone. The authors concluded that fluoxymesterone is an inferior choice for treating cancer-related anorexia and cachexia, whereas megestrol acetate and dexamethasone have similar appetite-stimulating effects but differing side effects.

Reviewing 15 published studies on the use of megestrol acetate for cancer-related anorexia and cachexia, Jatoi et al. (2000) found that this progestational agent improves appetite. However, only one study reported a significant improvement in the quality of life, while a second study demonstrated partial improvement. A third study noted an actual decline in the quality of life with megestrol acetate. Significantly, none of these 15 studies reported a survival advantage in patients receiving megestrol acetate. The authors were unable to reconcile the discrepancy between improvement in appetite and lack of improvement in the quality of life.

To elucidate further the mechanism of action of megestrol acetate, Reitmeier and Hartenstein (1990) treated 24 patients with this drug in dosages of 160 or 480 mg/day. All of these individuals had advanced cancer of varying primary sites; they were anorectic and had sustained severe weight loss before treatment with megestrol acetate. Body composition was determined by measuring bioelectrical impedance. Analysis with this technique showed a shift from fat to lean body mass in patients with unchanged weight, whereas patients with weight gain had an increase of both fat and lean body mass. As noted by the authors, weight gain due to treatment with megestrol acetate was caused by an increase in fat and body cell mass and was not due only to the accumulation of fluid.

Cachexia is a common problem of patients infected with the human immunodeficiency virus (HIV) and is indicative of a poor prognosis. Von Roenn et al. (1988) treated 14 patients with megestrol acetate if they were HIV positive, had lost more than 10 percent of their preillness body weight, and were losing weight at the time of enrollment in the study. Patients were given megestrol acetate in a dosage of 80 mg four times a day (total daily dose of 320 mg). All patients gained weight at an average rate of approximately 1.1 pounds per week. The average weight gain for the entire group was 14 pounds. Therapy with megestrol acetate was well tolerated. Peripheral edema, thromboembolism, and impotence did not occur. All patients reported a significant improvement in appetite while on therapy. In addition, 7 patients reported a marked improvement in their sense of well-being. Subsequent studies (Corcoran and Grinspoon 1999) have shown both appetite improvement and weight gain using 800 mg/day of megestrol acetate for HIV-related cachexia. Quality of life improved as well, but the weight gain was attributed mainly to increased fat mass.

A precautionary note on the use of megestrol acetate for AIDS-related cachexia was sounded by Henry et al. (1992). These investigators reported the development of insulin-dependent diabetes mellitus in a patient with AIDS 13 weeks after starting 320 mg of megestrol per day. When rechallenged with megestrol, the patient experienced an exacerbation of the diabetes. Until more information is available, the authors urged clinicians who manage patients with AIDS to be aware that megestrol acetate can induce a severe but reversible diabetic state and to use particular caution with patients who have a predisposition for pancreatitis or diabetes. In addition, Cushing syndrome, adrenal insufficiency, and hypogonadism may occur with the use of megestrol acetate (Corcoran and Grinspoon 1999).

Dronabinol. Interest has been renewed in the use of dronabinol (delta-9-tetrahydrocannabinol) as an appetite stimulant for patients with cancer. Wadleigh et al. (1990) studied 30 patients with unresectable cancer treated with oral dronabinol (delta-9-tetrahydrocannabinol in sesame oil). After a baseline observation period, patients were given dronabinol for up to six weeks at dosages of 2.5 mg once daily, 2.5 mg twice daily, or 5 mg once daily. Weekly weights were obtained, and each patient assessed appetite and mood on a visual analog scale. Five patients discontinued dronabinol because of adverse effects, and three stopped the drug due to progressive disease. Patients at all dosages continued to lose weight, although the rate of weight loss decreased with treatment at all dosages. Overall, improvement of symptoms was noted in both mood and appetite,

with 2.5 mg once daily being a no-effect dosage. Although the preliminary data are encouraging, more research is needed to delineate further
the role of this drug in the management of anorexia and cachexia.

Nutritional Problems

Many people with advanced cancer and other diseases experience alterations in taste perceptions, especially a reduction in the pleasant taste
of food and a bad taste sensation related to a specific food. This change
in food taste in turn leads to lessened appetite and decreased caloric intake. Negative taste sensations are most often associated with meat, cof-
fee, and chocolate (DeWys and Hoffman 1984).

Changes in taste compound the anorexia and cachexia syndrome.
Therefore, the goal of nutritional therapy at this stage is to improve the
quality and value of life (fig. 2.2). With or without pharmacologic inter-

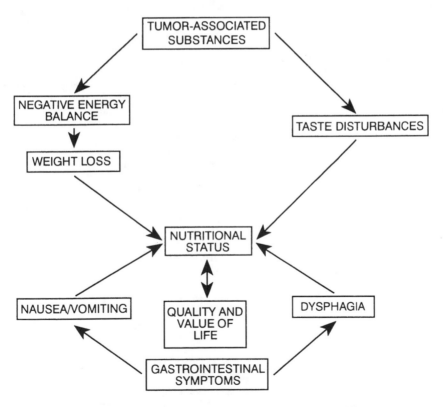

Figure 2.2.   Factors influencing a patient's nutritional status and quality of life

vention, the patient is allowed to eat whatever and whenever he or she desires. Because of the emotional connotation of food, families need to be reassured that dying loved ones want only enough food and drink to keep themselves comfortable. Indeed, McCann, Hall, and Groth-Juncker (1994) found that some terminally ill patients who preferred to refuse nutrition but felt obligated to eat to please their families suffered abdominal pain and nausea. Attempts to feed terminally ill patients artificially, particularly by the insertion of a nasogastric tube, are likely to add to distress rather than relieve it (Ashby and Stoffell 1991).

Hydration

The issue of hydration in the dying patient is less clear and more controversial than that of nutrition (table 2.3). For example, in the Letters to the Editor section of *Lancet*, Waller, Adunski, and Hershkowitz (1991) reported their experience with the hydration of patients dying within 48 hours. They compared two groups of 68 terminally ill cancer patients: one group of 13 patients (19%) received intravenous (IV) fluids, while

TABLE 2.3 Pros and Cons in the Use of Hydration for Terminally Ill Patients

---

Pro

    Dehydration and electrolyte imbalance may cause confusion, restlessness, and neuromuscular irritability.

    Dying patients are more comfortable if they receive hydration.

    There is no evidence that giving fluids alone may prolong life.

    Water is given to dying patients complaining of thirst, so why not administer parenteral fluids?

    Parenteral hydration is the minimum standard of care, and discontinuing this treatment breaks the bond with the patient.

    Withholding fluids from dying patients is too close to the edge of withholding therapies to other compromised patients.

Con

    Giving parenteral fluids may prolong the dying process.

    Less urine output means less need for bedpan, urinal, commode, or catheterization, and fewer bed-wetting episodes.

    There is less gastrointestinal secretion with fewer bouts of vomiting.

    There is less salivary gland fluid with diminished salivation and drooling.

    Less pulmonary secretion means less coughing, choking, pulmonary congestion, and death rattle.

    Edema and ascites are minimized.

    Diminished fluids and raised serum electrolyte levels may serve as a natural anesthetic to lessen the patient's level of consciousness.

    It is normal and more comfortable to die dehydrated.

Sources: Zerwekh (1987); Fainsinger and Bruera (1991); Lamerton (1991).

the second group was not given this treatment. The patients receiving IV fluids were treated at the request of their families. Blood urea nitrogen (BUN) and electrolyte levels were measured. BUN concentrations did not differ between patients receiving and those not receiving IV fluids. However, serum sodium levels were significantly lower in the IV-treated patients. Also, there was a significant association between the state of consciousness and serum sodium values, although the level of consciousness did not correlate with the administration of IV fluids. The investigators concluded that, since most of their patients had severe hydration and electrolyte imbalance, including those receiving IV fluids, decisions about treatment with IV fluids should be based on the preference of the patient and family. This report by Waller, Adunski, and Hershkowitz (1991) elicited a sharp rebuff from Lamerton (1991) several weeks later. Lamerton argued that, if a patient is hydrated before death, the bladder fills (causing urinary incontinence or distressing restlessness), the salivary glands produce excessive secretions and drooling, and the failing heart becomes overloaded (causing dyspnea and worsening the death rattle). Furthermore, Lamerton (1991) thought that, although electrolytes and IV therapy might impress the family, it is normal and more comfortable to die slightly dehydrated.

Zerwekh (1987), working as a hospice nurse, reported her observations of the beneficial effect of dehydration in the dying patient. She noted that with dehydration there was decreased urine output, which resulted in less need for the bedpan, urinal, commode, or catheterization and fewer episodes of bed-wetting. Gastrointestinal fluids were diminished, with fewer bouts of vomiting, and there was a reduction in pulmonary secretions, with less coughing and pulmonary congestion. As pulmonary secretions were diminished, patients who had difficulty swallowing experienced relief from choking and drowning sensations. Zerwekh also reported that reduced fluids and increased serum electrolytes served as a natural anesthesia to lessen the patient's level of consciousness. The opposite effects were seen in patients who died while receiving IV fluids. Finally, the major symptoms of dehydration were thirst and dry mouth, both of which were managed by small sips of oral fluids and good oral care.

In 1989, Andrews and Levine reported the results of a mail survey of hospice nurses in New Jersey and Pennsylvania. The questionnaire consisted of two major sections. The first section was related to experience and asked if the nurses had observed any patient in whom no food or fluid was given or taken for at least three days before death. The second section was a series of statements about dehydration to which the respondants were asked to rate their agreement on a five-point scale. Ninety-six of the 127 questionnaires were completed and returned, for a

76 percent response rate. Overall, the study showed that hospice nurses who were experienced in the matter of terminal dehydration viewed it as beneficial in the terminal stages of life. It was found that with dehydration there was a diminution of distressing symptoms such as choking, vomiting, and drowning sensations. Finally, hospice nurses reported that aggressive nutritional and hydration therapies were not essential to keep dying patients comfortable.

The perception expressed by nurses that terminal dehydration abates some distressing symptoms is not uniformly shared by physicians. In a survey of physicians in the United States, three-fourths would have used IV fluids at a sufficient rate to maintain hydration in a theoretical case of a comatose dying patient; only one-fourth would have opted for a judicious amount of fluid or no IV infusion. Half of the physicians mentioned IV fluids as part of the standard care of a dying patient. Thus, the use of IV fluids was often seen as "normal" in the terminally ill patient rather than as an extraordinary procedure for the treatment of hypercalcemia, hypoglycemia, and the like (Editorial 1986b). That this issue is not settled is underscored by the more recent comments of Fainsinger (1998), who noted that the data available are not adequate to justify any final conclusions regarding terminal hydration. Furthermore, he thought that there is a need for further definitive research and a careful individual assessment of the relevance of dehydration to each clinical situation.

Finally, Fainsinger and Bruera (1991) and Bruera and MacDonald (2000) advocated the use of hypodermoclysis (HDC) as an alternative to IV fluids for the dehydrated dying patient. HDC means the infusion of fluids into the subcutaneous space and offers many advantages over the IV route:

- Finding a venous access is unnecessary.
- HDC can be started by any staff member able to give a subcutaneous injection.
- HDC can be started and stopped without the needle clotting.
- Subcutaneous sites often last for days.

These investigators (Bruera et al. 1990) treated 58 patients with advanced cancer who required parenteral nutrition with HDC. There were 21 men and 37 women, with a mean age of 62 years. The reason for starting HDC was intestinal obstruction in 28 cases, nausea and vomiting in 10 cases, confusion in 14 cases, and dysphagia in 6 cases. HDC was administered using a no. 25 butterfly needle inserted underneath the skin of the anterior chest or abdominal wall. The needle was not changed until the site became symptomatic with pain, swelling, redness, or bleeding. A solution of two-thirds 5 percent dextrose and one-third saline was given at rates between 20 and 100 ml/hour. A total of 750 units of hyaluroni-dase, an enzyme that depolymerizes hyaluronic acid, causing a rapid diffusion of fluids subcutaneously, was added to each liter of solution. In addition, 20 to 40 mEq of potassium chloride was mixed in the solution, and in 38 cases morphine or hydromorphone was administered as well. The mean duration of infusion was 14 ± 9 days, with a mean volume of 1.3 ± 0.8 L/day. The mean dose of potassium chloride was 25 ± 8 mEq/L. HDC was discontinued because of death in 43 patients, oral hydration in 12 patients, and a need for fluid restrictions in 3 patients. Side effects were minimal: local infection (2 patients) and bruising (2 patients).

Constipation

Constipation is a common and often distressing symptom for patients with advanced disease. Although its etiology varies, constipation is generally associated with abdominal pain and discomfort, poor appetite, and ultimately impaired nutritional status. Additional complications include overflow diarrhea, confusion, urinary dysfunction, and nausea and vomiting (Fallon and O'Neill 1997).

NARCOTIC BOWEL SYNDROME

Drugs such as opioid analgesics, anticholinergics, and antidiarrheal agents may produce constipation. In 1984, Sandgren, McPhee, and Greenberger described the narcotic bowel syndrome (NBS) associated with the prolonged use or abuse of opioid analgesics in five patients. Clinical features of NBS included chronic abdominal pain, nausea and vomiting, abdominal distension, constipation, and at least one episode of intestinal pseudo-obstruction. These symptoms rapidly resolved in all patients when the administration of opioids was stopped.

Opioid analgesics affect gastrointestinal function through sigma receptors for muscle tone located throughout the gastrointestinal tract. Opioids reduce gastrointestinal motility, with an increase in muscle tone in the gastric atrium and first part of the duodenum. Gastric emptying is significantly delayed. Intestinal propulsive peristalsis is decreased while contractility and sphincter tone are enhanced. Lowered colonic motility as a result of opioids causes desiccated feces and constipation. Finally, opioids reduce gastric, biliary, and pancreatic secretions (Duthie and Nimmo 1987). Tolerance to the constipating effects of opioids often is absent or is slow to develop.

In an effort to delineate NBS in patients with advanced cancer, Bruera et al. (1987a) studied 191 patients treated with opioids between June

1985 and August 1986. All patients had metastatic disease without abdominal involvement, except 1 patient with liver metastases. Seven of the 191 (4%) were diagnosed as having NBS; all 7 had been receiving oral opioids, namely, morphine (3), hydromorphone (3), and levorphanol (1), for an average of 3 ± 2 months. The equivalent daily dose of oral morphine was 250 ± 170 mg. All patients developed severe bowel symptoms consistent with the diagnosis of NBS.

Hospitalization was required for management, including the use of parenteral analgesics. After metabolic abnormalities and mechanical intestinal obstruction were excluded, the patients were started on continuous subcutaneous infusions of metoclopramide (CSIM) at a dosage of 60 mg/day using disposable portable pumps. Metoclopramide was chosen because it is known to increase gastrointestinal motility. Significant improvements in nausea, vomiting, appetite, and abdominal distension were observed in all patients within 72 hours of the start of the infusion. The patients were subsequently returned to oral opioids. The CSIM was continued for 19 ± 6 days, with two patients being discharged home on this treatment. The CSIM was discontinued because of unrelated death (1 patient), return to oral metoclopramide (4 patients), cessation of opioids (1 patient), and toxicity (akathisia) after 14 days of infusion (1 patient).

NONDRUG ETIOLOGIES

In addition to drugs such as opioid analgesics, there are other possible etiologies for constipation. Intestinal obstruction, be it malignant or benign, is one possibility. Indeed, in reporting the experience in managing intestinal obstruction at St. Christopher's Hospice in London, Baines, Oliver, and Carter (1985) found that 13 percent of patients with malignant intestinal obstruction had constipation. Metabolic disorders such as hypercalcemia, hypokalemia, and uremia may also cause constipation. Autonomic failure in the form of the syndrome of cardiovascular autonomic insufficiency is another etiology for constipation (Bruera et al. 1986b). Occasionally a patient will present with constipation as one of the first signs of spinal cord or cauda equina compression from epidural metastases.

MANAGEMENT

After identifying and treating the underlying correctable causes, clinicians should encourage patients to increase their activity levels, especially ambulation, and oral intake of fluid. Barriers to defecation should be removed. Bedside commodes may be helpful for patients with limited ambulation. Most patients benefit from the addition of fiber to their diet. Excluding patients with intestinal obstruction, empiric therapy generally involves adding 3 to 4 grams of fiber to the daily diet and then gradually increasing this amount to 6 to 10 grams daily, as tolerated (Portenoy 1987).

Constipation may be prevented by anthraquinone cathartics (senna, cascara, danthron, and aloe). These drugs must undergo conversion to active metabolites in the colon and, therefore, are effective only in the distal colon. The anthraquinones act directly on the colon wall to stimulate peristalsis (Duthie and Nimmo 1987). Maguire, Yon, and Miller (1981) found that half a Senokot concentrated senna tablet (dose of 3.75 mg. of total sennosides) reversed the constipating effect of 60 mg of codeine or its equivalent. For optimal results, the senna derivative was taken together with the analgesic or on a similar schedule.

In a randomized, cross-over clinical trial, Sykes (1991) compared a mixture of equal proportions of lactulose and senna to codanthramer (not available in the United States) standard strength in 117 cancer patients with constipation. Patients with bowel diversion and evidence of intestinal obstruction were excluded. The lactulose-senna mixture produced a significantly greater frequency of stool than did codanthramer in patients receiving morphine and reduced the usage of suppositories and enemas. The incidence of diarrhea was greater with lactulose-senna; however, this generally dissipated with a 24-hour break and usually did not recur with the next dose. The patients' subjective assessment indicated that lactulose-senna was more likely than codanthramer to relieve constipation or to restore normalcy. Because increased doses of laxative were needed as the opioid doses increased, Sykes (1991) suggested that a schedule of laxative doses in relation to opioid doses may improve the effectiveness of laxative therapy over a system of ad hoc titration from a starting dose. Finally, a direct relationship between laxative and opioid doses was not observed, implying that opioids became relatively less constipating as the dosage was raised.

Other management for constipation includes the use of rectal agents and oral laxatives. Rectal agents include suppositories and enemas. Suppositories may contain glycerin alone, drawing fluid into the rectum and acting as a stimulant to defecation, or may contain an active drug such as bisacodyl. Enemas with tap water, saline, or soap suds may be used. Both suppositories and enemas are useful for the treatment of acute constipation or for the management of fecal impaction.

Oral cathartics include bulk-forming laxatives, lubricants, and osmotic (saline) cathartics. Bulk-forming laxatives, like bran, psyllium, and methycellulose, increase the stool bulk and soften its consistency by increasing the mass and water content of the stool. These agents are generally effective after two to four days of daily use. Of the lubricants, oral mineral oil is the preferred substance. This agent lubricates the stool, allowing for easier passage. In obtunded or confused patients, aspiration with a resultant lipoid pneumonia is a significant risk. This substance has little role in the management of chronic constipation but is useful in the acute treatment of fecal impaction or in acute transient constipation. Osmotic (saline) cathartics draw fluid into the bowel lumen, thereby decreasing the transit time of the stool. Magnesium salts, sodium salts, and lactulose are agents in this category. The use of magnesium and sodium salts is limited in patients with renal failure and congestive heart failure due to the systemic absorption of these ions. Generally the magnesium and sodium salts are effective for rapid evacuation within three to six hours. Lactulose is more effective for chronic use in dosages ranging from 15 to 30 ml, two to four times a day.

The contact cathartics are the primary agents used in the management of chronic constipation. These drugs cause increased mucosal secretion and a change in gastrointestinal motility. The docusates, anthraquinone, and diphenylmethane derivatives, as well as castor oil, are included in this category. Dioctyl sulfosuccinate is a docusate that is widely available and is often added as a stool softener to other contact cathartics. The diphenylmethane derivatives phenolphthalein and bisacodyl produce effects similar to those of the anthraquinones. Generally, they are safe and well tolerated for the management of constipation. The last of the contact cathartics is castor oil, but this agent is seldom used except in the management of acute, self-limited constipation (Portenoy 1987).

CENTRAL NERVOUS SYSTEM SYMPTOMS

Delirium

Delirium (acute confusional states) has been known and described since Hippocrates. It has been called "everyone's psychosis" or "reversible madness" and is one of the most commonly encountered mental disorders in general hospital practice. Indeed, it is estimated that approximately 10 percent of hospitalized medical and surgical patients are delirious at any given time (Lipowski 1987). The reported incidence of delirium in patients dying with cancer ranges from 53 to 85 percent (Massie, Holland, and Glass 1983; Bruera et al. 1987b).

By definition, delirium is a transient disorder of cognition and attention, one accompanied by disturbances of the sleep-wake cycle and psychomotor activity. It is classified as one of the organic brain syndromes.

Elderly patients are especially prone to delirium, and it has been associated with a high mortality. Self-injury of the patient is a serious risk, as are legal and ethical complications.

The cardinal clinical features of this syndrome are disorders of cognition and attention, disruption of the normal sleep-wake cycle, and either reduced or heightened activity and responsiveness. These symptoms develop acutely. They frequently fluctuate in severity during the day and are most pronounced at night.

Cognitive functions, mainly perception, thinking, and memory, are impaired to varying degrees. Disordered perception often results in confusion in addition to visual and auditory illusions. Thinking is disorganized and incoherent, which is evident in the patient's speech. Memory is impaired in all key aspects and orientation is usually defective, especially with regard to time. Attention (awareness, consciousness) is always disordered and attentional disturbances typically fluctuate during the day.

The normal sleep-wake cycle is disrupted. Often the patient sleeps or naps during the day, but at night he or she tends to be awake and agitated. This disorganized cycle appears to enhance the cognitive and attention deficits. Psychomotor behavior is altered in that the patient's movements and speech may be hypoactive or hyperactive. Hyperactivity is not a hallmark of delirium. Finally, emotions ranging from apathy or depression to fear or rage may also be present.

No specific diagnostic test for delirium is available, and the diagnosis is established on the basis of its essential clinical features. Cognitive and attentional symptoms are elicited and observed at the bedside. In general, the acute onset of cognitive and attention deficits and abnormalities, whose severity fluctuates during the day and tends to worsen at night, is practically diagnostic (Lipowski 1987).

Differentiating delirium from dementia is especially important and may be difficult when delirium is superimposed on preexisting dementia. A history of intellectual decline, occurring months or years before the onset of the acute cognitive disorder, is crucial for the differential diagnosis. In contrast to the delirious patient, the patient with dementia is usually alert and aware of the surroundings, fails to show fluctuating levels of awareness during the daytime, and shows defective knowledge of commonly known facts. The acute deterioration of cognitive and attentional functions in a patient known to have dementia suggests delirium (Lipowski 1989).

ETIOLOGIES

The occurrence of delirium in cancer patients is related to a wide range of causative factors, all of which can lead to diffuse cerebral dysfunction. Posner (1979) classified the neurologic complications of systemic cancer into the following areas: metastases to the nervous system, nonmetastatic involvement through metabolic encephalopathy (related to vital organ failure, electrolyte imbalance, and nutritional abnormalities), infections, vascular disorders, side effects of therapy (including use of opioid analgesics), and paraneoplastic syndromes. Subacute cerebellar degeneration, limbic encephalitis, and progressive multifocal leukoencephalopathy are types of remote effects of tumor or paraneoplastic syndromes that may present with dementia early in the course of the disease or may even precede the diagnosis of cancer. It is important, therefore, for clinicians to recognize and diagnose these entities, since delirium may be superimposed on the process.

To understand better this syndrome of delirium in patients dying of cancer, Massie, Holland, and Glass (1983) studied 13 patients with cancer who died during hospitalization. Eleven of the 13 (85%) developed delirium as measured by a standardized delirium scale. Typically, the delirium developed as the illness progressed and appeared most frequently when the patient was near death. In 2 of the 11 patients it was not possible to discover the cause, since no laboratory tests were performed. In all of the remaining cases (9), delirium was attributed to metabolic encephalopathy, structural invasion of the brain by tumor, or a combination. Factors identified as causing the metabolic encephalopathy were the failure of a vital organ (such as kidney, liver, or lung), toxic levels of opioids, electrolyte imbalance, and sepsis. In more than half of the patients, the metabolic encephalopathy was due in part to increasing doses of opioid analgesics. In this study, it was difficult to establish a single cause for delirium in patients with advanced cancer.

In a less controlled study, Bruera et al. (1987b) retrospectively reviewed the cases of 30 consecutive patients who died after being admitted to the hospital for at least one week under their care. All the patients had metastatic cancer. Unlike the study by Massie, Holland, and Glass (1983), this study did not use a standardized delirium scale. The diagnosis of delirium was made clinically in the presence of a confusional state with or without hallucinations or hyperactivity. Sixteen of the 30 patients (53%) developed delirium, by the authors' definition, more than 48 hours before death. In only 2 of these cases (13%) was a cause found, and in both it was related to drug therapy (amitriptyline and morphine). Also, improvement was noted in both these cases after either discontinuation or change in drug treatment.

In a larger study, Lawlor et al. (2000) prospectively studied 104 patients with advanced cancer admitted to an acute palliative care unit in a university-affiliated teaching hospital. They found a very high rate of delirium in these patients: 42 percent in patients on admission, 45 percent for first onset after admission, and 88 percent in patients who died. Delirium was reversible in 46 (49%) of 94 episodes in 71 patients. Psychoactive drugs, predominantly opioids, and dehydration were associated with reversibility, while hypoxic encephalopathy and metabolic factors were not associated with reversibility. The authors concluded that delirium is a frequent, multifactorial complication for patients with advanced cancer. Despite its terminal presentation, delirium is reversible in about 50 percent of the episodes and therefore warrants a search for underlying, correctable causes such as psychoactive medications and dehydration. Change of opioid, dose reduction, or stopping other psychoactive drugs, and hydration frequently reverses this delirium.

Stedeford and Regnard (1991) provided a systematic scheme for assessing delirium in patients with advanced cancer (table 2.4). Reduced alertness is common in acute confusional states. Opioid analgesics are

TABLE 2.4   The Symptoms and Causes of Delirium

Symptoms
  Memory failure
  Changed alertness
  Impaired concentration
  Abnormal experiences
  Altered behavior
  Mood disturbance
Causes
  Drugs
    Opioids
    Corticosteroids
    Antidepressants
    Nonsteroidal anti-inflammatories
  Infection
    Respiratory
    Urinary
  Metabolic disturbances
    Hypercalcemia
    Hyponatremia
    Uremia
  Cardiac or pulmonary disease
  Brain disease
    Metastases
  Trauma
    Subdural hematoma
    Impacted bone fracture
  Treatable anxiety or depression
  Unrelated psychiatric illness

Source: Stedeford and Regnard (1991).

frequently blamed, but they are an unlikely cause in a patient receiving them chronically. Commonly overlooked drugs include corticosteroids, nonsteroidal anti-inflammatory drugs, and antidepressants. Infections, especially respiratory and urinary, may change alertness, as will metabolic alterations such as hypercalcemia, hyponatremia, and uremia. The presence of underlying cardiac or pulmonary disease may cause hypoxia accompanied by increased alertness and marked anxiety.

An unsuspected subdural hematoma or an impacted bone fracture may reduce alertness and cause confusion. Finally, abnormal experiences and hallucinations are infrequently related to the use of morphine. Tolerance to this side effect may occur.

Management

Once the diagnosis of delirium is made, the following guidelines may be useful in the management of this syndrome (Levine, Silberfarb, and Lipowski 1978; Massie, Holland, and Glass 1983; Lipowski 1987, 1989; Stedeford and Regnard 1991; Lawlor et al. 2000):

- If the clinician suspects metabolic encephalopathy secondary to opioid analgesic use, he or she should change the opioid used. Avoid polypharmacy, since drugs other than opioids have also been implicated.
- If dehydration is present, consider hydration using hypodermoclysis (HDC).
- Provide measures to help reduce anxiety, agitation, and disorientation. These may include a quiet, well-lit room with a few familiar objects and a visible calendar and clock. Short but frequent contacts with a supportive person, preferably a family member, help alleviate the disorientation. Good nursing care is crucial for orienting and reassuring the patient.
- The impaired ability to function mentally is very distressing to patients who are acutely aware of it. Depression, with possible risk of suicide, must be kept in mind due to the patient's poor impulse control.
- Sedation may be necessary to relieve severe agitation, disruptive behavior, or insomnia. Haloperidol is usually the safest and most effective drug for this purpose. Massie, Holland, and Glass (1983) suggested that the intramuscular injection of 0.5 to 2 mg reduces agitation without causing sedation or hypotension. Doses, repeated at 30-to 60-minute intervals, are then titrated against behavior. Extrapyramidal signs are controlled by benzotropine, 2 mg twice a day. The authors also recommended changing the patient to an oral dose

as soon as possible, at three-quarters of the level of the intramuscular dose. For lesser degrees of disturbed behavior, they suggested the use of 1 mg of haloperidol, 1 to 2 mg of trifluoperazine, or 10 to 25 mg of thioridazine given orally twice daily.

- Involvement of a psychiatrist to help interpret the situation for the family and collaborate with the staff in the management of the patient is useful.

Depression

Psychological problems, especially depression, are often assumed to be common in cancer patients. Despite the recent advances in the treatment of cancer, the diagnosis is still terrifying to patients and families. Their initial reaction is generally shock and denial. Patients may complain of feeling depressed, anxious, and irritable. They may experience a loss of appetite and insomnia during the first 7 to 10 days after the diagnosis. This acute stress response is considered normal and is usually resolved when treatment is started. For some patients, however, these symptoms persist and may interfere with medical management.

DIAGNOSIS

Apart from the acute stress response, reactive depression is the most frequent psychological problem diagnosed in patients with cancer (Holland 1987). Depending on the method of diagnosis employed, the prevalence rate for depression in these individuals seems to be between 23 and 58 percent (Brown et al. 1986). However, many of these studies were flawed by the use of biased samples or reliance on self-report instruments.

In an effort to identify psychological problems in cancer patients, the Psychosocial Collaborative Oncology Group (PSYCOG) studied 215 randomly accessed patients from three major cancer treatment centers (Derogatis et al. 1983). Each patient was evaluated by a common protocol comprising a formal psychiatric interview and standardized psychological tests. The American Psychiatric Association's *Diagnostic and Statistical Manual of Mental Disorders* (DSM-III) was used in making the diagnosis. The prevalence rate of mental disorders among the cancer patients was high, at 47 percent.

The authors noted that this is about twice the rate usually found in medical patients and three times as high as prevalence rates reported for the general population. However, the most frequent diagnoses were adjustment disorders, which accounted for 68 percent of the psychiatric diagnoses. These adjustment disorders consisted of varying elements of anxiety and depression and were attributed to the stress of the diagnosis of cancer. Thirteen percent had a major depression, 8 percent had organic mental disorders related to analgesics or metabolic abnormalities, 7 percent had personality disorders that predated the illness, and 4 percent of those patients with a positive psychiatric condition were experiencing a disorder with depression or anxiety as the central symptom.

Another major finding of the PSYCOG study was that most of the psychiatric disorders found in the sample of cancer patients can be successfully treated. In addition, the fact that most (53%) of these patients did not have any psychiatric disorder revealed by a careful diagnostic interview should not be ignored. Despite the terror commonly associated with cancer, most patients are able to mobilize their psychological resources in a normal, reasonably adaptive way (Glass 1983).

In a more recent review, Cody (1990) suggested that adjustment disorders are common, observed in some 25 to 35 percent of patients. Only a small minority, approximately 5 to 15 percent, became seriously depressed, which, she felt, dispels the myth that depression is an inevitable reaction to a terminal illness. However, the prevalence of depression is higher in cancer patients with the greatest disability and distressing physical symptoms, especially uncontrolled pain (Pirl and Roth 1999).

Clinical symptoms, such as anorexia, weight loss, and fatigue, are common to both cancer and depression and therefore are of little value in diagnosing depression in the cancer patient. Thus, the diagnosis must rely heavily on psychological symptoms, such as the presence of dysphoric mood (sadness, anxiety) and feelings of hopelessness, helplessness, and worthlessness. The differentiation between reactive depression and major depression is often difficult, as these two diagnoses represent a continuum of severity of depressive symptoms rather than two separate diagnostic categories.

Cancer patients at high risk for developing depression include those with poor pain control; a more deteriorated physical condition; advanced stages of disease, especially pancreatic cancer; and a history of prior depression or psychiatric illness (Holland 1987).

Depression and Suicide

In 1986, Brown et al. studied 44 terminally ill patients from the palliative care service at St. Boniface General Hospital, in Winnipeg, Manitoba, to determine if suicidal thinking was a normal finding in dying patients. Among these 44 patients, the majority (34) had never wished death to come early. Of the remaining 10 patients, 3 were or had been suicidal and 7 more were found to have clinical depressive illness. The authors thought that suicidal thoughts and desires for death appeared to be linked exclusively to the presence of a mental disorder. Furthermore, generalizing their findings, the authors postulated that patients with terminal illness who are not mentally ill are no more likely than the general population to wish for premature death.

In a related article, Breitbart (1987) reviewed the topic of suicide in cancer patients. Few systematic studies have been done to determine the true incidence of cancer suicide; however, these studies do suggest that, although relatively few cancer patients commit suicide, they are at increased risk. The frequency of passive suicide and the degree of treatment noncompliance or refusal, which represents a deliberate decision to end life, are unknown, and the actual incidence of suicide in cancer patients may be underestimated. Men with cancer are at increased risk of suicide compared to the general population. The most common method of suicide in the cancer patient is a medication overdose of either sleep or pain drugs. According to Breitbart, factors in the vulnerability to suicide with cancer are advanced illness and poor prognosis, delirium, loss of control and helplessness, preexisting psychopathology, prior and family history of suicide, exhaustion, and fatigue.

Finally, Ripamonti et al. (1999) showed that suicide among terminally ill cancer patients is rare. From September 1985 to December 1997, they evaluated suicides in all patients with terminal cancer cared for at home by 12 associated palliative care teams organized in Milan and its province. Of the 17,964 patients, only 5 cases of suicide (0.027%) were recorded. Two patients jumped out of a window, two shot themselves, and one took an overdose of morphine. The authors speculated that continuing treatment of symptoms and psychological support given to these patients may reduce the risk of suicide.

MANAGEMENT

The treatment of depression may include short-term supportive psychotherapy and psychopharmacologic drugs. Short-term supportive psychotherapy is generally effective for patients with a normal response to stress or an adjustment disorder. This mode of treatment is based on a crisis intervention model, and 4 to 10 sessions are generally sufficient to reduce symptoms to a tolerable level. The inclusion of a family member or close friend in these sessions has been found to be helpful. Group sessions with patients who share the same problem are an alternative approach (Holland 1987).

Prolonged or severe symptoms indicate the presence of a major depression, which should be managed with a combined regimen of supportive psychotherapy and psychopharmacologic drugs.

The tricyclic antidepressants have been the mainstay in the treatment

TABLE 2.5   The Side Effects of Antidepressant Drugs

Drug	Sedation	Insomnia	Anticholinergic Effects	Orthostatic Hypotension	Nausea	Usual Daily Oral Dose (mg)
Tricyclic anti- depressants						
Amitriptyline	+++	0	+++	++	0	75–150
Imipramine	++	0	+++	+++	0	75–150
Doxepin	+++	0	++	+++	0	75–150
Nortriptyline	++	0	+	+	0	100–150
Selective serotonin reuptake inhibitors						
Sertraline	0	++	0	0	++	50–100
Fluoxetine	0	++	0	0	++	20–40
Paroxetine	0	++	0	0	++	20–40
Other drugs						
Trazodone	+++	0	+	++	+	150–250
Maprotiline	++	0	+	++	0	50–75
Amoxapine	++	0	+	++	0	100–150
Alprazolam	+	0	0	0	0	1.5

Sources: Holland (1987); Cody (1990); Potter, Rudorfer, and Manji (1991); Block (2000).

Note: 0 = no side effect; + = minor side effect; ++ = moderate side effect; +++ = major side effect.

of depression (Holland 1987; Cody 1990). They are also useful in the management of neuropathic pain, which is independent of their effect on mood. Amitriptyline, imipramine, doxepin, and nortriptyline are most commonly prescribed. With cancer patients and patients with other terminal illnesses, treatment is generally empiric because of the paucity of good scientific data from randomized clinical trials.

The tricyclic antidepressants have generally equivalent clinical efficacy and differ only in the intensity of side effects (table 2.5). The choice of antidepressants is usually dictated by the patient's clinical state. Depressed patients with agitation, anxiety, and insomnia usually welcome the sedative properties of drugs such as amitriptyline, whereas patients with psychomotor retardation respond better to the activating drugs such as imipramine.

The main side effect of the tricyclic antidepressants is their effect on the cardiovascular system, namely, delay in cardiac conduction or arrhythmia (Potter, Rudorfer, and Manji 1991), and orthostatic hypotension. Anticholinergic side effects are often bothersome, especially dry mouth, blurred vision, hesitancy of micturition, urinary retention, and constipation. Patients already receiving opioids may experience a worsening of dry mouth and constipation. Over time, a tolerance to these unwanted side effects seems to develop (Cody 1990).

For poorly understood reasons, patients with cancer or other chronic disease seem to respond to lower doses than do otherwise physically normal patients. In practice, it is best to tailor the dose to the response and the severity of side effects. Amitriptyline, for example, is started at 10 to 20 mg/day given at bedtime and increased by 25 mg every one or two days until a beneficial effect occurs. Generally, all antidepressants take two to three weeks to exert their antidepressant effect, although patients may benefit from the anxiolytic or sedative effect much earlier.

The clinician should consider second-generation antidepressants (trazodone, maprotiline, amoxapine, and alprazolam) for patients not responding to the tricyclic antidepressants or for those who cannot tolerate the side effects of anticholinergic drugs. This generation of drugs, however, has not been shown to be superior to the tricyclic antidepressants in terms of antidepressant effects.

In one of the few randomized clinical trials in this area, Holland et al. (1991) compared alprazolam to progressive muscle relaxation in cancer patients with anxiety and depressive symptoms. One hundred forty-seven cancer patients were randomized to receive either alprazolam, 0.5 mg three times a day, or a progressive muscle-relaxation technique over a ten-day period. Seventy patients were randomized to drug and 77 to relaxation. Four measures of anxiety and depression were used. Both treatment arms resulted in a significant decrease in observer- and patient-reported anxious and depressed symptoms. Although both treatments were effective, patients receiving alprazolam showed a slightly more rapid decrease in anxiety and a greater reduction of depressive symptoms. Based on their study, the investigators recommended the use of alprazolam and relaxation for cancer patients experiencing symptoms of anxiety and depression.

The third-generation antidepressants, the selective serotonin reuptake inhibitors (SSRIs), are as safe and effective as the tricyclic antidepressants for depression. Although there are no controlled trials in terminal illnesses, the SSRIs (sertraline, fluoxetine, and paroxetine) are often the first-line drugs for the treatment of depression in dying patients when immediate onset of action is not essential. In general, paroxetine and sertraline are better tolerated by terminally ill patients because they have fewer active metabolites that can accumulate and cause unwanted toxicity (Block 2000). The role of psychostimulants, such as methylphenidate and dextroamphetamine, in managing depression continues to evolve. For patients with a limited life expectancy, these drugs can reduce the distress of the patient and the family and create opportunities for them to cope more effectively with the dying process. Patients who are extremely debilitated and fatigued may experience an improvement in energy and mood within 24 hours of starting treatment. The psychostimulants are best used by patients who have weeks or several months to live (Block 2000).

Finally, antidepressants of the monoamine oxidase inhibitor class are not suitable for depressed cancer and terminally ill patients because of the necessity for dietary restrictions (Cody 1990).

SYSTEMIC SYMPTOMS

Dyspnea

Dyspnea, or shortness of breath, is a distressing symptom to both the patient and the family. In 1974, Wilkes reported dyspnea as one of the ten major symptoms after admission to a small 25-bed unit especially interested in caring for the dying patient. Reuben and Mor (1986a) reviewed the epidemiology of dyspnea occurring in terminally ill cancer patients during the last six weeks of life. This study found dyspnea to be more common in these patients (70.2%) than had previously been appreciated. In addition, the severity of the symptom was at least moderate in more than 28 percent of patients who were able to grade their dyspnea. In 1989, Higginson and McCarthy reported that, near death, 21 percent of their patients developed dyspnea as the main symptom. Furthermore, this became the most common severe symptom at death.

Dyspnea with Malignant Disease

Lung cancer is the leading cause of cancer death in men and women in the United States. It is not surprising that the presence of this disease correlates highly with the symptom of dyspnea. The pathophysiology producing shortness of breath in patients with lung cancer includes the following:

- endobronchial or central lesions causing obstruction resulting in atelectasis or pneumonia;
- parenchymal replacement by tumor to the extent that a restrictive ventilatory defect occurs;
- diffuse lymphangitic spread of the tumor throughout the lungs;
- phrenic nerve paralysis from compression by mediastinal lymph node metastases leading to impaired diaphragmatic function;
- pleural effusions resulting in reduced lung capacity;
- superior vena caval syndrome.

Dyspnea may occur by differing mechanisms in patients with pulmonary metastases. For example, the sudden onset of shortness of breath in patients with known parenchymal disease suggests the development of an associated effusion, bleeding into a metastasis with sudden subpleural expansion, or the occurrence of a pneumothorax. Likewise, the onset of increasing dyspnea associated with cough and debilitation often denotes lymphangitic carcinomatosis despite a normal chest radiograph (Pass and Roth 1987). Thus, like pain, dyspnea must be evaluated on an ongoing periodic basis to monitor any changes, be they subtle or obvious.

Finally, other factors can cause or contribute to the clinical symptom of dyspnea, such as the following:

- prior cancer treatment with surgery (postpneumonectomy), radiation therapy (postradiation pulmonary fibrosis), or chemotherapy (e.g., the use of bleomycin);
- generalized debility of terminal disease;
- pulmonary embolism;
- aspiration pneumonia;
- the presence of underlying disease, especially chronic obstructive pulmonary disease and congestive heart failure;
- massive ascites compromising pulmonary function; and
- anxiety, which frequently can enhance dyspnea during attacks of breathlessness (Higginson and McCarthy 1989) (Table 2.6).

DYSPNEA WITH NONMALIGNANT DISEASES

Nonmalignant advanced diseases can cause dyspnea (table 2.7). Chronic progressive cardiac and respiratory diseases frequently end with terminal dyspnea. Aspiration pneumonia is often missed as a cause of shortness of breath, as it may occur silently during sleep in conditions in which esophagopharyngeal muscle tone is impaired, as in motor neuron disease or systemic sclerosis. Deformity of the chest wall causing dyspnea may be the consequence of prior poliomyelitis, kyphoscoliosis, or ankylosing spondylitis. Chronic intercostal or diaphragmatic weakness may result from motor neuron disease. Finally, the chronic use of drugs can cause dyspnea through diffuse lung injury (Regnard and Ahmedzai 1991).

MANAGEMENT

As with the management of pain and other symptoms in the dying patient, the clinician should seek etiologies for dyspnea and, when these are

TABLE 2.6   The Causes of Dyspnea in Patients with Advanced
Cancer

Carcinoma of the lung
   Obstructing lesions with atelectasis and pneumonia
   Restrictive ventilatory defect
   Lymphangitic spread
   Metastases
   Impaired diaphragmatic function
   Pleural effusions
   Superior vena caval syndrome
   Bleeding
   Pneumothorax
Prior cancer therapy
   Postpneumonectomy
   Postradiation fibrosis
   Chemotherapy
Generalized debility
Thrombotic pulmonary embolism
Tumor pulmonary embolism
Aspiration pneumonia
Pneumonia due to infection
Underlying chronic obstructive pulmonary disease or congestive
     heart failure
Massive ascites
Anxiety

Sources: Pass and Roth (1987); Higginson and McCarthy (1989).

identified, take corrective action. For example, bronchodilators can be helpful in relieving symptomatic bronchospasm. Saunders (1982) outlined a group of drugs useful in the management of dyspnea. Corticosteroids may be used in the management of mediastinal lymph node compression resulting from superior vena caval obstruction, lymphangitic carcinomatosis of the lung, and bronchospasm. Antibiotics are recommended on an individual basis rather than being administered routinely. Factors such as the symptoms caused by the pneumonia and the patient's age, overall condition, and respiratory capacity should be considered. If antibiotics are not justified, then symptoms can be controlled by the use of opioids and anticholenergic drugs such as scopolamine. In a study (Volicer et al. 1986) of 40 patients with Alzheimer disease, 62 percent were not treated with antibiotics if they developed symptoms of pneumonia. The authors of the study thought that the treatment of infections with antibiotics did not necessarily increase patients' comfort. Furthermore, the authors did not favor empiric antibiotic therapy without a work-up and stated that the patients' comfort was maintained by the frequent use of analgesics and antipyretics.

TABLE 2.7 The Causes of Dyspnea in Patients with Advanced Nonmalignant Disease

---

Chronic obstructive pulmonary disease
  Congestive heart failure
  Infection
Chronic congestive heart failure
Aspiration pneumonia
Recurrent pulmonary embolism
Chest wall deformity
Intercostal or diaphragmatic weakness
Anemia
Drugs

Source: Regnard and Ahmedzai (1991).

Small doses (5 to 10 mg every four hours) of morphine effectively relieve dyspnea. Morphine is known to decrease the ventilatory response to carbon dioxide, hypoxia, and exercise and to diminish oxygen consumption at rest and during exercise in normal persons. Morphine also reduces the respiratory rate and the sensation of gasping for air or air hunger (Cooke 1989). As with pain control, the clinician should titrate the dose against the response and increase it as needed. Tranquilizers, such as chlorpromazine (Walsh 1993) or diazepam (Davis 1997), may be added to manage the anxiety associated with dyspnea. Hoskin and Hanks (1988) reported their experience with advanced cancer patients admitted to the Continuing Care Unit at the Royal Marsden Hospital, in London. They found that the prime indication for morphine in 22 percent of patients was for the relief of respiratory symptoms rather than pain. Finally, current evidence does not support the use of nebulized morphine for the relief of dyspnea (Davis 1997).

A small bedside fan is often effective in managing terminal dyspnea (Kerr 1989). Preferably, the fan is placed to propel fresh air from an open window across the patient's face. This stream of cool air stimulates temperature and mechanical receptors of the facial trigeminal nerve in the cheek, thus altering the perception of breathlessness. Trigeminal nerve receptors also line the nasopharynx, and this may explain why some patients experience relief of dyspnea from the use of nasal oxygen.

The accumulation of excessive pulmonary secretions when the patient is dying, the so-called death rattle, is quite disturbing for families and staff. Generally, this can be managed with scopolamine in doses of 0.4 to 0.6 mg given every four to eight hours as required (Saunders 1982; Cooke 1989). Saunders (1982) also recommended administering concomitant morphine, 10 to 15 mg, to increase sedation and prevent the occasional central nervous system excitement caused by scopolamine. In the study by Hoskin and Hanks (1988), scopolamine by injection was given with diamorphine to ameliorate respiratory symptoms from retained pulmonary secretion in 34 percent of their patients. One patient received a four-day infusion. When scopolamine was administered by injection, the median number of injections required was 1, with a mean of 3.6 and a range of 1 to 20.

Saunders (1982) suggested that oxygen can be useful in acute dyspnea but that better control of chronic dyspnea can be achieved with opioids. Supplemental oxygen should be used with care in patients with chronic obstructive pulmonary disease, who may retain carbon dioxide. Kerr (1989), however, questioned the necessity of using oxygen in the dyspneic dying patient. He pointed out the occurrence of a bedside medical melodrama with all attention focused on the oxygen, its flow rate, and placement of the cannula. On the other hand, a 1993 publication by Bruera et al. demonstrated a beneficial effect of oxygen delivered at 5 L/min. via mask in terminally ill cancer patients with hypoxia and dyspnea at rest. In view of the uncertainty surrounding the use of oxygen, Davis (1997) suggested a 24-hour trial of continuous or intermittent oxygen via a cannula accompanied by subjective assessment and pulse oximetry, if possible. If the trial is successful, then relatively long term use is appropriate (table 2.8).

In patients with large pleural effusions, rapid relief of dyspnea occurs after the removal of the pleural fluid. Evidence suggests that this improvement in breathing is due to a reduction in the thoracic cage size, which allows the inspiratory muscles to operate more efficiently (Es-

TABLE 2.8   Pros and Cons in the Use of Oxygen

Pro

    Reverse hypoxia. One study demonstrated a beneficial effect of oxygen delivered at 5 L/min via mask in terminal cancer patients with hypoxia and dyspnea at rest.

    Placebo effect for the patient and the family.

    A 24-hour trial of continuous or intermittent oxygen via a cannula is appropriate and should be accompanied by subjective patient assessment and, if possible, pulse oximetry.

Con

    The occurrence of a medical melodrama with all the attention focused on the oxygen, its flow rate, and the placement of the cannula.

    Potential loss of respiratory drive, especially in patients with chronic obstructive pulmonary disease who may retain carbon dioxide.

    Difficulty in talking and dry mouth.

Sources: Kerr (1989); Davis (1997).

tenne, Yernault, and DeTroyer 1983). Thus, in the dyspneic patient with a pleural effusion, a therapeutic thoracocentesis is reasonable and may result in clinical improvement.

Finally, coughing often accompanies the shortness of breath. Expectorants, which increase the volume of sputum, are generally not helpful. Mucolytic drugs, such as acetylcysteine, reduce the viscosity of bronchial secretions and occasionally are useful. For patients on opioid analgesics for pain control, escalating the dosage is often effective in suppressing the cough as well.

Given this array of therapeutic interventions for the management of dyspnea, it is quite interesting that Higginson and McCarthy (1989) concluded from their study that these treatments are generally ineffective. Using a standardized measurement instrument, symptom assessment scores for patients with dyspnea showed no change over time despite a variety of treatments. According to the authors, uncontrolled dyspnea appears to need greater research attention.

Urinary Incontinence

The involuntary loss of urine or urinary incontinence is a clinical problem that has often been overlooked and is poorly understood. In a study by Wilkes (1974), incontinence was one of the ten major symptoms after admission in 296 patients cared for in a small, 25-bed palliative care unit in England. In this same study, urinary incontinence was the reason for admission to respite care in 11 percent of the cases.

As reviewed by the Consensus Conference on Urinary Incontinence in Adults (1989), continence requires a compliant bladder and active sphincteric mechanisms such that maximal urethral pressure always exceeds intravesical pressure. Normally, voiding requires sustained and coordinated relaxation of the sphincters and contraction of the urinary bladder. These functions are regulated by the central nervous system through both autonomic and somatic nerves. This system requires the integration of visceral and somatic muscle function and involves control by voluntary mechanisms originating in the cerebral cortex. These voluntary mechanisms are learned and culturally prescribed (i.e., toilet training).

ETIOLOGIES

Incontinence can be produced by any pathologic, anatomic, or physiologic factor that disrupts the pressure gradient between the bladder and the urethra. In the general adult population, the most common clinical forms of urinary incontinence are stress incontinence, urge incontinence, overflow incontinence, and a mixed form. In stress incontinence, dysfunction of the bladder outlet causes a leakage of urine as intraabdominal pressure is raised above urethral resistance while coughing, bending, or lifting heavy objects. Stress incontinence has many etiologies, including direct anatomic damage to the urethral sphincter.

Urge incontinence occurs when a person senses the urge to void but is unable to inhibit leakage long enough to reach the toilet. In most cases, inhibited bladder contractions contribute to the incontinence. In patients with advanced cancer, central nervous system involvement by primary brain tumors or metastatic lesions may cause urgency leading to incontinence. Also, bladder tumors or other cancers involving the bladder may cause local irritations, which often are manifested as urgency (Herwig 1980).

Overflow incontinence occurs when the bladder is unable to empty normally and becomes overly distended, leading to frequent urine loss. Lesions in the true pelvis involving the peripheral pelvic nerves can often cause overflow incontinence. Any factor that causes outflow obstruction, such as direct invasion of the bladder by a cancer, can lead to uncontrolled loss of urine due to overflow. Also, the mechanical effects of fecal impaction often lead to overflowing incontinence (Wrenn 1989).

Many types of urinary incontinence fall into the mixed category, displaying various aspects of more than one of the major subtypes. Occasionally a urinary fistula, such as vesicovaginal, presents with incontinence in patients with extensive pelvic cancer. As a result of radical pelvic surgery, spinal cord compression below T11, damage to the sacral plexus, or an episode of outlet obstruction, a hypotonic bladder may develop. Features include difficulty in starting micturition, an intermittent stream, incomplete emptying, stress incontinence, persistent dribbling incontinence, and repeated infections (Regnard and Mannix 1991).

The term *functional incontinence* is applied to those patients in whom the function of the lower urinary tract is intact but other factors such as immobility or severe cognitive impairment result in urinary incontinence. This category is highly applicable to chronically ill patients.

In occasional circumstances, urinary incontinence may be related to prior cancer therapy. For example, treatment with cyclophosphamide can cause bladder wall fibrosis, leading to pronounced contraction of the bladder and loss of compliance. Radiation therapy has a similar effect (Herwig 1980).

It is clear that urinary incontinence is caused by multiple, often interacting factors. It is important for the clinician to identify the reversible conditions such as infection, delirium, and drugs.

As with other symptoms in the dying patient, a clinical evaluation for possible etiologies of urinary incontinence is of paramount importance.

The patient should not be relegated to the discomfort of an indwelling catheter until correctable conditions have been thoroughly explored. A careful history and physical examination with special attention to the preillness voiding pattern often produce an accurate diagnosis. Simple laboratory measurements, including urinalysis, serum creatinine or blood urea nitrogen (BUN) levels, urine cultures, and postvoid residual urine volume, may be clinically helpful.

MANAGEMENT

The management of urinary incontinence in terminally ill cancer patients generally includes the use of drugs and protective devices. Behavior therapy, while highly successful in areas such as nursing homes, has limited use in terminal care because of the time necessary to train patients in these techniques.

The pharmacologic therapies currently used in the management of urinary incontinence have not been studied in well-designed clinical trials. Nonetheless, it has been suggested that many agents are beneficial for patients with urge incontinence due to uninhibited contractions of the bladder outlet muscle. Since these drugs increase the bladder's capacity, they may precipitate the retention of urine. Bladder relaxants include the anticholinergics, direct smooth muscle relaxants, calcium channel blockers, and imipramine.

Alpha-adrenergic agonists act as stimulants on the bladder outlet. These drugs produce smooth muscle contraction at the bladder outlet and may improve stress incontinence.

Protective devices available include absorbent pads or garments, indwelling catheters, and external collection devices such as condom catheters. Absorbent pads or garments are convenient temporary devices but are not suitable for long-term use. For men, external collection devices may be useful but are associated with an increased incidence of urinary tract infection. Practical external collection devices for women are not generally available (Consensus Conference 1989).

Chronic indwelling catheters, which are often necessary in the terminal setting, invariably lead to urinary tract and systemic infections. Herwig (1980) thought that self-catheterization, when possible, is more physiologic and is better tolerated by the patient. Intermittent catheterization is the treatment of choice for patients with a hypotonic bladder (Regnard and Mannix 1991). Whatever the cause, urinary incontinence is managed by catheterization, whether self-, intermittent, or continuous, as death nears (Woodruff 1997).

Pressure Sores

Pressure sores or decubitus ulcers are a serious problem for the hospitalized or homebound bedridden patient. The prevalence of this problem ranges from 3 to 11 percent. The in-hospital mortality rate of patients with pressure sores is between 23 and 37 percent (Allman 1989). Complications include osteomyelitis and sepsis. Hanson et al. (1991) reported a 13 percent incidence of pressure sores among hospice patients, with more than half (62%) occurring within two weeks of death. Because dying patients are chronically bedridden, the occurrence of pressure sores adversely influences the quality of life and, thus, prevention of this problem is of utmost importance.

The term *decubitus ulcer* (derived from the Latin word *ducub,* meaning "lying down") is often used to describe this problem. However, this is a misnomer, since a large number of these sores develop while the patient is in a sitting position (Reuler and Cooney 1981). Therefore, the term *pressure sore* is more accurate and describes the underlying pathophysiology.

Etiologies

Although many factors contribute to the development of pressure sores, four have been identified as critical: pressure, shearing forces, friction, and moisture. Pressure is the essential element. In the skin, the normal internal capillary pressure is 32 mm Hg. When external pressures greater than this amount are applied, the skin capillaries as well as the lymphatics collapse, leading to significant disruption of blood and lymphatic flow. The net result of this heightened pressure is time dependent. A pressure of 70 mm Hg applied for more than two hours produces irreversible tissue damage; if the same pressure is applied repeatedly for five minutes alternating with five minutes of no pressure, few changes occur. External pressures are higher in areas where soft tissue overlies bony prominences. Therefore, the great majority of pressure sores are located in the lower part of the body, with the sacral and coccygeal areas, ischial tuberosities, and greater trochanter accounting for the majority of sites of pressure sores.

Shearing forces are another causative factor in the development of sores. Clinically, these forces are working when the head of the bed is raised, causing the body to slide down, transmitting pressure to the sacrum and deep fascia. At the same time, the posterior sacral skin is fixed, because of friction with the bed, and shearing forces in the deep part of the superficial fascia lead to stretching and distortion of blood vessels, which causes thrombosis and undermining of the dermis.

Friction is the force generated when two surfaces in contact move across each other, as when a patient is dragged across the bedsheets. Friction removes the outer protective layer of skin, accelerating the onset of ulceration. The final critical factor is moisture, caused by fecal or urinary leakage or perspiration, increasing the risk of pressure sore formation fivefold (Reuler and Cooney 1981).

RISK FACTORS

Although pressure, shearing forces, friction, and moisture are the causes of pressure sores, other factors place a patient at risk for developing this problem. To further define those factors associated with the presence of a pressure sore among adult patients hospitalized at Johns Hopkins Hospital, Allman et al. (1986) studied one group of patients with pressure sores and another group of patients at risk. The group at risk were patients who had been or were expected to be confined to a bed or chair for at least one week. Among 634 adult patients, 30 (5%) had a pressure sore and 78 (12%) were at risk. Furthermore, cancer was the only variable noted significantly more often among patients at risk. Comparing the patients with sores to the patients at risk, the authors found that fecal incontinence, diarrhea, fracture, use of urinary catheters, decreased weight, dementia, and hypoalbuminemia were associated with having a pressure sore. In addition, the authors reported that the presence of hypoalbuminemia, fecal incontinence, and fractures helped to identify bedridden patients at greater risk for developing pressure sores.

In a more didactic and less scientific fashion, Duffield (1989) listed both intrinsic and extrinsic factors predisposing to the development of pressure sores. Intrinsic factors are old age, debility, immobility, sedation or impaired consciousness, loss of sensory or motor function, spasticity, emaciation or obesity, malnutrition (especially vitamin C and protein), anemia, fever, edema, peripheral vascular disease, urinary and fecal incontinence, dehydration, and electrolyte imbalance. Extrinsic factors include loss of the skin's natural acidity (soap, laundry, or bed linen) or bacteria (disinfectants); repeated injections at vulnerable sites; poor nursing technique (e.g., body contact with impervious plastic); and systemic corticosteroids, nonsteroidal anti-inflammatory drugs, and chemotherapy and radiation therapy (table 2.9).

PREVENTION

The old adage "an ounce of prevention is worth a pound of cure" certainly applies to the area of pressure sores. In 1987, Colburn suggested a

TABLE 2.9   Risk Factors for Developing
Pressure Sores

Immobility
Elderly age
Nutritional deficiency, especially vitamin C
Age-related skin changes
Urinary and fecal incontinence
Diarrhea
Hypoalbuminemia
Pressure of a fracture
Dementia
Sedation or impaired consciousness
Loss of sensory or motor function
Emaciation or obesity
Anemia
Fever
Edema
Peripheral vascular disease
Dehydration
Electrolyte imbalance
Repeat injections at vulnerable sites
Poor nursing techniques
Drugs
Chemotherapy and radiation therapy
Pain

Sources: Allman (1989); Duffield (1989); Ryan
(1989).

preventive strategy for pressure sores in hospice patients, which includes
the following:

- relieving pressure, especially over all bony prominences;
- maintaining the skin's integrity by keeping the skin clean and as free
  as possible from contamination with urine and feces;
- improving nutritional status by correcting nutritional deficiencies
  and promoting adequate hydration;
- promoting patient movement by providing active and passive motion
  as well as frequent turning;
- educating the patient and family regarding the need for a prevention program and the family's role.

Clearly, the dictum "where there is no pressure, there is no sore" must
not be forgotten (Reuler and Cooney 1981).

MANAGEMENT

Once a pressure sore occurs, management varies widely, often depending on local preference. Multiple topical therapies (Vohra and McCollum 1994), various antipressure devices, and specialized beds have been advocated on the basis of uncontrolled, observational studies. In a randomized clinical trial, Allman et al. (1987) compared the use of airfluidized beds to conventional therapy for pressure sores in hospitalized patients. Air-fluidized beds contain ceramic beads covered by a closely woven polyester sheet. Pressurized, warm air is forced up through the beads, which take on the characteristics of a fluid. Patients float on the bed without pressure on bony prominences. Other benefits include a dry environment, a freely movable surface, and a bacteriostatic bead system. Patients allocated to conventional therapy were to be repositioned at least every two hours, permitted to use heel and elbow protectors, and placed on a vinyl alternating air mattress covered by a 19-mm thick foam pad. The air mattress was placed on top of the regular hospital bed. Patients assigned to air-fluidized beds were to be repositioned every four hours. In both groups, physicians were allowed to order a plastic surgery consult, topical treatment with saline or povidone-iodine, enzymatic debridement with a combination preparation of fibrinolysin and deoxyribonuclease, sterile gauze dressings, and whirlpool therapy as needed. Thirty-one patients were randomized to the air-fluidized bed, and 34 patients received conventional care. Overall, the results showed that the air-fluidized beds are more effective than conventional therapy, especially for large sores. The use of the air-fluidized bed was associated with a significant reduction from the baseline in both the intensity of the pain and the level of discomfort. In addition, the authors emphasized the need to determine the effectiveness of air-fluidized beds in long-term care settings.

Clark et al. (1990) reported an unusual complication with the use of air-fluidized beds, namely, concealed bleeding. They described two cases in which blood drained rapidly into the chamber of an air-fluidized bed. This hemorrhaging was not obvious, since no signs of blood were detected on the patient's dressing or bed surface. To monitor for occult blood loss with air-fluidized beds, they recommended the use of a latex sheet.

PROGNOSIS

It is very difficult to determine the prognosis for the healing of pressure sores. As a general rule, patients in the last few weeks of life who are deteriorating rapidly (deterioration noticed daily) are unlikely to show healing of anything but the most minor skin damage, and even wound cleansing may be incomplete. Slower deterioration (weekly) may allow some partial healing of shallow ulcers (<0.5 cm) if nutrition is adequate. Slow deterioration (monthly) may allow time to clean and heal deep ulcers (>0.5 cm) (Bale and Regnard 1989).

Summary

Nausea and vomiting are problems encountered frequently in dying patients. Indeed, one study (Reuben and Mor 1986b) found that 62 percent of terminally ill cancer patients experienced nausea and vomiting at some time during their last two months of life. In addition, these investigators reported that only one-third of the nauseated patients had received an antiemetic prescription. The implication of this study is clear: physicians must better appreciate the impact of this symptom on the quality of life of dying patients and must manage it more aggressively. If a correctable cause, such as hypercalcemia, is identified, then it should be treated appropriately. If an uncorrectable cause, such as metastatic liver disease, is found, then every attempt must be made to control this problem using antiemetic drugs and/or nonpharmacologic interventions.

About one-half of patients with advanced cancer (Curtis, Krech, and Walsh 1991) and other disease experience anorexia that results in cachexia. Corticosteroids have been used widely for years to manage this anorexia-cachexia syndrome, but there is no sound, scientific support for this practice. Multiple studies have shown that corticosteroids can improve appetite and the patient's sense of overall well-being; however, no study reported weight gain. In addition, these drugs are not without side effects, which may compound existing problems, such as weakness and confusion.

Megestrol acetate offers promise for the management of anorexia and cachexia in patients with cancer and AIDS. Its exact mechanism of action is unknown, but it seems to be an appetite stimulant, and weight gain is due not to the accumulation of excess fluid but rather to increases in fat and body cell mass. The optimal dosage of megestrol acetate to stimulate appetite is 800 mg per day. However, treatment with megestrol acetate is not inexpensive: an 800-mg dose costs $20–25.

Nutrition and hydration are two very emotion-laded problems associated with the management of dying patients. With advanced disease, the patient's taste perception is negatively altered, especially in regard to meat and sweets. Since the goal of nutritional therapy at this point is to improve the quality and value of life, the patient should be allowed to eat whenever and whatever she or he desires. To avoid conflict, the physician should reassure the family that dying patients want only enough food and water to keep themselves comfortable.

The issue of hydration is less clear cut than that of nutrition. One group, predominantly physicians, feels that parenteral hydration, be it by the intravenous or the subcutaneous route, is the minimal standard of care for the dying patient. Nurses, on the other hand, generally espouse a different opinion, namely, that terminal hydration only enhances the body's secretions, which in turn causes a more painful death. The clinician must recognize both sides of this argument. A patient's dying without all the trappings of parenteral fluids and without excessive pulmonary and gastrointestinal secretions is both more comfortable for the patient and more humane for the caregiver. To help the patient reach this end, the physician must spend time with the patient and family, discussing the hydration issue and reassuring them that the lack of parenteral fluids does not represent abandonment by the physician and that death with dehydration is painless.

Constipation is a common and often distressing problem for patients with advanced disease. Although the etiology varies, a correctable cause, such as electrolyte imbalance, should be investigated and managed appropriately. The narcotic bowel syndrome is unusual; if it is diagnosed, a trial of continuous subcutaneous infusion of metoclopramide should be started. The prevention of constipation is of utmost importance; to this end, high-fiber diets, ambulation, increased oral fluids, and the removal of barriers to defecation are encouraged. In addition, the routine administration of laxatives, such as senna or a mixture of senna and lactulose, on a schedule similar to that for opioid analgesics is effective.

The reported incidence of delirium in dying cancer patients ranges from 53 to 85 percent. As with other symptoms, a reversible etiology should be sought and managed. One study found delirium to be correctable in approximately 50 percent of the episodes (Lawlor et al. 2000). Polypharmacy is often overlooked in this setting. If sedation is required, haloperidol is the preferred drug.

Despite the common misperception, serious depression is distinctly unusual in dying patients (5 to 15%). It can be treated with short-term supportive psychotherapy and psychopharmacologic drugs, such as the tricyclic antidepressants or the selective serotonin reuptake inhibitors. Alprazolam, a second-generation antidepressant, is useful for patients with anxiety associated with depressive symptoms. The great majority of dying patients do not wish for early death, and suicide in dying patients is rare.

Dyspnea is the most common severe symptom before death. Modest doses of morphine (5 to 10 mg every four hours) effectively relieve this symptom, as can the use of a small bedside fan. Antibiotics and supplemental oxygen are infrequently indicated. Occasionally, thoracocentesis provides transient relief of symptoms if a large pleural effusion is present. Excessive pulmonary secretions ("death rattle") are best managed with scopolamine (0.4 to 0.6 mg given every four to eight hours as required) along with morphine. Coughing, which occasionally accompanies shortness of breath, is best treated by escalating the dosage of opioids.

Urinary incontinence is an infrequent but troublesome problem in the care of dying patients. Just before death, this is managed by protective devices such as indwelling or condom catheters.

Approximately one in five dying patients develops pressure sores, and few of these heal. Simple measures, including good skin care, frequent positioning, and, if available, the use of air-fluidized beds, are effective in making patients more comfortable.

Chapter 3

Other Problems of Patients with Cancer

Malignant Intestinal Obstruction

Intestinal obstruction is a common clinical problem for patients with advanced cancer, particularly those with colorectal or ovarian cancer. When cancer recurs or extends in the form of either large or small bowel obstruction, medical management can be difficult because of the associated psychosocial issues. On one hand, the clinical picture often is characterized by a patient unable to eat and malnourished, with intermittent abdominal discomfort and pain, who has received extensive prior cancer treatment, including surgery, radiation therapy, and chemotherapy. In view of these factors, the patient presents a poor risk for surgical intervention. On the other hand, the patient's family becomes increasingly frustrated at watching their loved one "waste away" because of an inability to sustain any significant nutrition. This, in turn, leads to intense pressure on the physician to "do something." With few exceptions, clinical situations like this one sharply focus on the question of the quality of life.

Etiologies

The exact incidence of intestinal obstruction in hospice patients is not known, but investigators from St. Christopher's Hospice in London estimated that 3 percent of all their patients had intestinal obstruction (Baines, Oliver, and Carter 1985). This escalated to 10 percent in patients with colorectal carcinoma. This obstruction is frequently related to extrinsic pressure from extramural masses rather than tumor recurrence within the bowel lumen. These extramural masses usually arise from serosal metastases or implants on the small bowel or may be due to metastatic involvement of the omentum, peritoneum, or other abdominal structures. The result is that these extramural metastases adhere to several loops of bowel, which accounts for the clinical observation that multiple sites of obstruction are common in these patients. However, nonmalignant causes of obstruction can occur. Osteen et al. (1980) retrospectively reviewed 66 cases in which the patient developed intestinal obstruction after treatment for cancer. In 32 percent of these patients, a benign cause of intestinal obstruction was found, such as adhesions, internal hernias, or radiation enteritis. In the 62 percent for whom obstruction was due to malignant neoplasm, the following risk factors were identified: a prior diagnosis of colorectal carcinoma, the presence of known metastatic disease, advanced stage of the primary tumor at diagnosis, and a short interval since the initial treatment of the cancer.

Advanced ovarian carcinoma ranks second in tumor sites causing intestinal obstruction. Krebs and Goplerud (1983) studied bowel obstruction in advanced ovarian carcinoma in 98 patients. They devised a risk score for these patients and identified the following significant negative prognostic factors: age greater than 65 years, poor nutrition, liver involvement or distant metastases, severe ascites, unsuccessful combination drug therapy, and previous radiation therapy to the whole abdomen. Although the colorectum and ovary are the most common primary sites, other areas, including gastric organs, pancreas, urinary tract, cervix, endometrium, skin, peritoneum, breast, and lung, have been reported (Osteen et al. 1980; Aranha, Folk, and Greenlee 1981; Baines, Oliver, and Carter 1985; Turnbull, Guerra, and Starnes 1989).

Significant insight into the problem of malignant intestinal obstruction, including management, was provided by Baines, Oliver, and Carter (1985). They studied 40 patients with intestinal obstruction treated at St. Christopher's Hospice in London. The patients were 26 to 94 years old, with a mean age of 59. Thirty-eight were managed without surgery; their symptoms included nausea and vomiting (100%); abdominal pain caused by hepatomegaly, tumor masses, or distension (92%); intestinal colic or crampy abdominal pain (76%); diarrhea (34%); and constipation (13%). This study highlights the spectrum of clinical symptoms associated with intestinal obstruction. In addition, symptoms such as crampy abdominal pain and distension may be intermittent, because the obstruction may be incomplete at initial presentation.

MANAGEMENT

The initial management of the patient with bowel obstruction is surgical evaluation. There are few patients who are found to have only a single obstructing lesion or whose previous operative findings do not preclude surgery. For the majority of cases, surgical intervention is not feasible because of the presence of multiple sites of obstruction and the overall poor clinical condition of the patient. At this point, general medical management consists of the insertion of a nasogastric (NG) tube for suction and intravenous (IV) fluids to maintain electrolyte and fluid balance. Using this approach, Osteen et al. (1980) reported a 23 percent rate of spontaneous resolution. This resolution occurred quickly, and there seemed to be little benefit in extending the NG suction beyond three days. Unfortunately, this approach provided only a temporary solution, since 41 percent eventually required surgical decompression.

Of the 40 patients managed in St. Christopher's Hospice (Baines, Oliver, and Carter 1985), 92 percent had undergone surgery, predominantly a bypass procedure, at least once. For only 2 of these patients was further surgical intervention possible to relieve the obstructive symptoms. The remaining 38 were managed without surgery and without the discomfort of prolonged NG suction and IV fluids.

The authors evaluated the response to their treatment regimens based on the severity of symptoms before treatment, the dosage of medication necessary to control symptoms, and the frequency of medication needed to maintain control. Smooth muscle–relaxant drugs, such as loperamide, scopolamine, and atropine, completely controlled crampy abdominal pain in 68 percent of the patients.

In well over half of the patients, scopolamine or atropine was given by subcutaneous (SC) continuous infusion. In patients with abdominal pain related to hepatomegaly, tumor masses, or distension, 89 percent were rendered pain-free with varying regimens of morphine, oxycodone, and diamorphine (not available in the United States). Again, SC continuous infusions, especially with diamorphine, were employed. Nausea and vomiting, however, were more difficult to control: for only 13 percent of the patients were these symptoms completely controlled.

The most effective antiemetic drugs were phenothiazines (prochlorperazine, chlorpromazine) and butyrophenones (haloperidol). The SC continuous infusion route was also used with haloperidol. Patients were encouraged to eat and drink liberally, and dehydration was not a problem. Diarrhea was controlled in 56 percent with loperamide and codeine. Constipation occurred in few patients, and it was treated with stool softener for those patients in whom a single rectal or colonic obstruction was suspected.

Not surprisingly, the survival time for the 38 patients treated without surgery was short—a mean of 3.7 months. This, however, is similar to other reported survival times (Osteen et al. 1980; Aranha, Folk, and Greenlee 1981; Krebs and Goplerud 1983). For example, Osteen et al. (1980) reported a median survival of 3.0 months after operation for 32 patients found to have obstructions by recurrent cancer. In the group of 20 patients with a nonmalignant cause of obstruction, 9 (45%) died of recurrent cancer, with a median survival time of 5.5 months after surgery.

A study from the Pain Therapy and Palliative Care Division of the National Cancer Institute of Milan (Ventafridda et al. 1990a) also demonstrated the effectiveness of this type of conservative management. Twenty-two inoperable symptomatic patients with malignant intestinal obstruction were managed with continuous SC or IV infusions of morphine, haloperidol, and scopolamine. Morphine, for pain, was started with an initial dose of 0.5 mg/kg, and the final range was 20 to 80 mg/day. Scopolamine, for crampy pain and hypersecretions, was instituted at a dose of 1 mg/kg, and the final range was 40 to 380 mg/day. Haloperidol was given for nausea and vomiting at a beginning dose of 0.05 mg/kg, and the final range was 2 to 15 mg/day. All drugs were given via an infusion pump. The mean age of the patients was 58 years, with a range of 40 to 80 years. The treatment lasted 2 to 50 days, with a mean of 13.4 days. Seventeen patients were treated at home, and 5 were treated in the hospital. In all cases, the continuous infusions were continued until death. Because of this approach, an NG tube with suction was avoided in 19 of the 22 patients. For the remaining 3 patients with upper intestinal obstruction due to gastric, pancreatic, and hepatic cancers, it was necessary to insert an NG tube because therapy with antiemetic drugs was ineffective. IV fluids were administered to only 1 patient to relieve thirst. For the 21 other patients, thirst and dry mouth were managed by oral fluids, ice cubes, pieces of pineapple, or chewing gum. The investigators noted that the use of IV fluids raises the volume of gastrointestinal secretions and therefore increases vomiting. An analysis of the patients' self-descriptive records showed that, after two days of treatment, the pain score decreased by more than 80 percent from the initial value. Based on their experience, the authors concluded that, for terminally ill cancer patients, pain and vomiting from inoperable intestinal obstruction, excepting obstruction of the upper bowel, can be controlled with continuous parenteral infusions of analgesic and antiemetic drugs, in the hospital and at home, without recourse to the placement of an NG tube or to IV hydration.

Octreotide is often used if continuous infusions of analgesic and antiemetic drugs are ineffective (Baines 1997). Octreotide is a synthetic polypeptide analog of somatostatin which inhibits secretion of growth hormone, gastrin, secretin, vasoactive intestinal peptide, pancreatic polypeptide, insulin, and glucagon. It also blocks the secretion of gastric acid, pepsin, pancreatic enzymes, bicarbonate, and intestinal epithelial water and electrolytes. At doses of 150 to 300 µg SC, or IM twice daily, or 300 to 600 µg via 24-hour continuous infusion, octreotide is effective, especially if a large volume of vomitus is present. In one study, octreotide eliminated, in approximately three days (range of 1 to 6 days), nausea and vomiting for all patients for whom it was tried and significantly decreased the volume of NG drainage (Abrahm 2000). Although dexamethasone, in doses of 8 to 60 mg per day, has been reported to improve intestinal obstruction by decreasing peritumor edema, there is limited scientific evidence of its efficacy (Baumrucker 1998).

Problems with hydration appear to be related to the level of intestinal obstruction. Distal bowel obstruction (rectum, colon, and ileum) still provides sufficient mucosal surface area for fluid absorption to prevent symptomatic dehydration. More proximal bowel obstructions may cause mild symptoms such as a dry mouth, which can be treated by ice chips, oral fluids, and the like. Obstructions proximal to the midjejunum may require parenteral fluids to treat symptomatic dehydration, especially thirst. The majority of patients, however, do not require IV hydration. Obstructions in the duodenum or proximal jejunum cause gastric retention, with associated epigastric discomfort and large-volume vomiting. If this obstruction is partial and motility is impaired, the patient may be helped with metoclopramide. If obstruction is complete, however, NG suction is occasionally required. As the patient's condition deteriorates, dehydration results in reduced vomiting, decreases pulmonary secretions, and lessens urinary incontinence. Dehydration is normal at the end of life (Regnard 1988).

Malignant Dysphagia

Dysphagia, or difficulty in swallowing, is a problem not infrequently encountered in dying patients. Sykes, Carter, and Baines (1988) described this symptom as a presenting complaint in 11.7 percent of the terminally ill patients they studied. The clinical consequences of dysphagia are malnutrition and dehydration, which often lead to conflict regarding management.

There are many possible etiologies for the symptom dysphagia, since the act of swallowing involves not only the gastrointestinal tract from the oropharynx to the lower esophagus but also brainstem control of this function. As a practical matter, dysphagia in the cancer patient is generally related to primary tumors in the head and neck, esophagus, and upper stomach, in addition to tumors that metastasize to lymph nodes in the mediastinum, causing external compression.

ETIOLOGIES

Sykes, Carter, and Baines (1988), from St. Christopher's Hospice and the Royal Marsden Hospital in London, retrospectively reviewed their experience with dysphagia in patients with terminal malignant disease. This symptom was identified in 92 of 797 consecutive patients admitted over a 15-month period. The severity of dysphagia was assessed according to the consistency of food that caused symptoms, from firm solids to liquids. The perceived level of obstruction, the presence and location of any associated pain, and symptoms of oral dryness or soreness were also noted. Excluding the 42 patients who died within one week, 33 patients had objective evidence of dysphagia on assessment, whereas the remaining 17 had no clear-cut evidence of dysphagia on assessment. The majority of patients in this latter group had tumors remote from the upper gastrointestinal tract and presented with significantly less severe dysphagia than the 33 patients with clinical confirmation of this symptom. The esophagus was the leading primary site (30%) in patients with clinical evidence of dysphagia, followed by stomach (15%), oropharynx (12%), non-Hodgkin lymphoma (10%), tongue (6%), and miscellaneous (15%). More than half of the patients were able to describe a roughly consistent region, either above or below the clavicles, where food or liquids seemed to stick. In addition, one-third of the patients complained of pain or discomfort in the same area. Most patients had difficulty swallowing soft solids and liquids of varying consistencies. Twenty-one of these 33 patients were examined by limited symptom-directed autopsy. Local obstruction in the upper gastrointestinal tract by primary, metastatic, or multifocal tumor was found in 81 percent. Multiple obstructions were present in four patients. Of the patients who had identified the level of the obstruction (i.e., above or below the clavicles), their descriptions were confirmed 92 percent of the time. The survival of these dysphagic patients did not differ significantly from the hospice average.

Although Sykes, Carter, and Baines (1988) demonstrated that almost all patients in their study with objective evidence of dysphagia after careful assessment had local obstructive disease due to tumor, there are etiologies for this symptom in addition to tumor compression. It is generally assumed that infection of the oral cavity with the fungus *Candida albicans* can cause dysphagia as well as other oral symptoms; however, Finlay (1986) questioned this relationship. Mouth swabs were taken at weekly intervals in 140 consecutive patients in the Strathcarron Hospice in England. Patients were queried regarding the presence or absence of a wide variety of oral symptoms. Dysphagia was reported in 21 percent of patients with positive *Candida* cultures and in 32 percent of patients for whom the culture was negative for *Candida*. This difference was not statistically significant. Also, no correlation was shown between *Candida* and other mouth symptoms except between white lesions of the mouth and positive *Candida* cultures. Finlay concluded that the results of this study do not confirm that oral *Candida* is associated with symptoms or signs in the mouth, although oral candidiasis is common among terminally ill patients. Oral *Candida* and symptoms were not affected by antifungal treatment with nystatin. The author surmised that infection with *C. albicans* may be the result rather than the cause of mouth problems, indicating that general oral hygiene is more important than antifungal therapy.

In 1982, Carter, Pittam, and Tanner studied, both clinically and pathologically, a group of 17 terminally ill patients with advanced squamous cell carcinoma of the head and neck. More than half of these patients had combined clinical and pathologic evidence of perineural spread, and the incidence of nerve involvement detected morphologically was high (88%). Clinically, sensory changes predominated, with multiple nerve involvement occurring in one-third of the patients. The most important conclusion to emerge from this study was the identification of an apparently new dysphagia syndrome in patients with advanced carcinoma of the oropharynx. The clinical picture was one of complete or nearly complete mechanical obstruction, but little or no direct block was found at autopsy. The signs and symptoms were due to perineural invasion into the ipsilateral vagal trunk, variable involvement of the sympathetic chain, splinting of the pharynx by local fibrosis, and tumor in the soft tissue of the neck. The resultant effect was neuromuscular incoordination producing dysphagia. As emphasized by the authors, the recognition of this syndrome is important because short-term palliation can be achieved with dexamethasone, 8 mg daily.

MANAGEMENT

In the study by Sykes, Carter, and Baines (1988), all of the 33 patients with clinical evidence of organic dysphagia were treated conservatively. This management included the following:

- dietary intervention to ensure a diet of the right consistency for each patient;
- strict maintenance of oral hygiene;
- pain control by standard treatments such as morphine and antiemetic drugs as required;
- the use of dexamethasone, generally 4 to 12 mg daily, if the tumor was likely to respond or when an external obstruction from nodal metastases was present; and
- the occasional use of palliative radiation therapy.

The response to treatment was assessed for each patient. Overall, 58 percent of patients showed a response to treatment, from complete resolution to improved intake of food of the same consistency. The most refractory dysphagia occurred in patients with combined primary and metastatic tumor. Only 3 of the 33 patients were thought to have died other than completely peacefully. NG intubation, parenteral feeding, and feeding gastrostomy were not used in this study. Although these techniques ensure adequate caloric intake, two of them are restrictive and none prevents the aspiration of saliva. Rather than adding worthwhile life at this stage of the disease, they may prolong an uncomfortable death.

Two techniques clinically relevant to the treatment of malignant dysphagia are intracavitary irradiation and endoscopic laser palliation. Forty patients with advanced carcinoma of the esophagus and gastric cardia received palliative therapy by intracavitary irradiation. As reported by Rowland and Pagliero (1985), 65 percent experienced relief of dysphagia. In a study from the Mayo Clinic, Ahlquist et al. (1987) were able to improve swallowing in approximately 80 percent of the 25 patients with advanced esophageal cancer treated with endoscopic laser therapy. A single laser treatment provided adequate palliation for more than half the patients until the time of death. Furthermore, no laser-related mortality or major morbidity occurred.

Barr and Krasner (1991) reported their experience with endoscopic laser therapy in 40 patients with obstructing gastric and esophageal cancer causing dysphagia. The patients' swallowing ability significantly improved with laser therapy, and 58 percent of the patients died at home. The mean survival was 16 weeks.

The endoscopic insertion of esophageal stents has provided significant palliation for patients with malignant dysphagia. Self-expanding metallic stents cause fewer complications than plastic stents. Furthermore, endoscopic laser therapy has a lower rate of complications than either plastic or self-expanding metallic stents. Thus, the recommended endoscopic approach for palliating malignant dysphagia includes laser therapy or the insertion of self-expanding metallic stents (Van Dam and Brugge 1999).

Neuromuscular Dysfunction

Weakness, defined as a deficiency in strength or power, is a common symptom in terminal illness and is present in the vast majority of patients with advanced cancer. As noted by Lichter (1990), weakness in terminal illness may be related to neuromuscular disorders from a wide variety of etiologies (table 3.1). Also, other forms of neuromuscular dysfunction are occasionally encountered in patients with advanced cancer.

Etiologies

Several well-known (paraneoplastic) syndromes demonstrate the remote effects of cancer on neuromuscular function (Bunn and Ridgway

TABLE 3.1   The Neuromuscular Causes of Weakness
in Terminal Illness

Related to the Cancer	Unrelated to the Cancer
Nervous system damage by tumor to:	Transient ischemic attacks
	Motor neuron disease
Brain	Myasthenia gravis
Spinal cord	Parkinsonism
Peripheral nerves	Peripheral neuropathies due to:
Carcinomatous neuropathy	Diabetes mellitus
Myopathy	Nutritional disorders
	Alcoholism
	Systemic diseases

Source: Lichter (1990).

1989). Patients with either dermatomyositis or polymyositis have five to
seven times the incidence of malignant neoplasm compared to the general population. Clinically, this syndrome is characterized by a gradually
progressive muscular weakness occurring over a period of weeks to
months. The weakness eventually stabilizes, is usually not disabling, and
usually involves the proximal muscles. In the majority of cases, the my-
opathy and cancer present within one year of each other. The myasthenic
syndrome (Eaton-Lambert) is another classic example of a cancer, most
often small cell carcinoma of the lung, producing a remote or paraneoplastic effect on the neuromuscular system. This myasthenic syndrome is
characterized by muscle weakness and fatigue, which are most pronounced in the pelvic girdle and thigh. Other common features include
dryness of the mouth, dysphagia, dysarthria, and peripheral paresthesia.
Successful treatment of the underlying small cell lung cancer can produce improvement in the muscular symptoms. Finally, the association of
myasthenia gravis and thymoma is well established. Patients with myasthenia gravis present with muscular weakness, especially in the ocular and
cranial muscles. There is a tendency for fluctuation and partial reversibility by cholinergic drugs. A number of tumors, including lym-
phomas and those of the pancreas, breast, prostate, ovary, thyroid, cervix,
kidney, rectum, and palate, have been described in association with myasthenia gravis, but the incidence is the same as that expected in the normal population.

   Bruera et al. (1988a), from the Cross Cancer Institute in Edmonton,
Alberta, prospectively studied 61 consecutive patients with advanced
breast cancer to assess muscle electrophysiology. This group of patients
was compared to 20 normal age-and sex-matched female controls. Nutritional status, lean body mass, voluntary and involuntary muscle electro-

physiology tests of the adductor pollicis, and ultrasonographic measurement of the triceps brachialis, sternomastoid, and adductor pollicis muscles were determined in patients and controls. Patients with breast cancer were chosen because the incidence of malnutrition is significantly lower in this population than in patients with other cancers, such as lung or gastrointestinal. Malnutrition alone has been reported as a cause of abnormal muscle electrophysiology. The function of the adductor pollicis muscle of the hand was assessed because people with advanced cancer still use their hands, as compared to muscles of the upper or lower limbs, which tend to atrophy with disuse. In addition, tumor mass and Karnofsky performance status were determined in the patient group.

The nutritional status and the lean body mass did not differ significantly between patients and controls. Also, ultrasound studies of the three muscle groups failed to reveal any difference between patients and controls. There was, however, a difference in the muscle electrophysiology tests, with the cancer patients demonstrating abnormalities. These abnormalities were not correlated with tumor mass, performance status, the site of the primary breast cancer (right versus left), the use of chemotherapy known to cause nerve damage (vincristine), or the number of courses of chemotherapy.

The authors concluded that they were unable to determine by their study the reason for the abnormal muscle electrophysiology in the patients with advanced breast cancer. They emphasized the importance of more research in this area as well as the major role that this muscular dysfunction may play in producing clinical symptoms such as weakness.

Muscle Cramps

Muscle cramps generally have been regarded as a nuisance but benign, whatever the clinical setting. This perception was challenged by Steiner and Siegal (1989), who prospectively studied 50 cancer patients with new complaints of muscle cramps. Cramps were defined as localized, painful, involuntary skeletal muscle contractions of sudden onset. All patients were evaluated with a detailed neurologic examination and extensive laboratory and radiologic studies. The 50 patients included 36 women and 14 men who ranged in age from 12 to 80 years. The majority of patients had solid tumors, with the breast as the most frequent site. Most patients had frequent attacks that commonly occurred in both arms and legs. Nocturnal cramps were described by slightly more than half of the patients.

For 41 patients (82%), a specific neural, muscular, or biochemical abnormality was identified as the most likely etiology of muscle cramps. Most abnormalities were related to the peripheral nervous system. Muscle disease and biochemical abnormalities infrequently caused cramps.

The use of amitriptyline resulted in a peripheral neuropathy in one case. For 9 patients (18%), no identifiable pathologic condition could be established. For two-thirds of the patients, muscle cramps were the first symptom of a previously unrecognized pathologic process.

Muscle cramps in cancer patients should not be ignored and frequently highlight the presence of an identifiable neurologic disorder (Steiner and Siegal 1989). Furthermore, the use of simple clinical and laboratory measures often leads to a diagnosis in the majority of patients.

Malignant Ulceration

Although the occurrence of malignant ulceration in patients with advanced and uncontrolled cancer is not especially common (8%) (Hockley, Dunlop, and Davies 1988), it is very distressing to both the patient and the family. The disagreeable odor of these large, fungating tumors often deepens the patient's sense of helplessness, embarrassment, and social isolation.

Etiologies

Wood (1980) categorized the location of malignant ulceration by anatomic site, namely, head and neck, thorax, perineum, abdomen, and extremities. Head and neck lesions are frequently of squamous cell origin and are especially difficult to treat. Generally, these patients have been treated with surgery, radiation therapy, and chemotherapy before the disease recurs. Complications of large, fungating head and neck tumors include airway obstruction and the invasion of major blood vessels with the possibility of erosion and fatal hemorrhage. A tracheostomy may be required to maintain an open airway. Lesions overlaying the carotid artery occasionally erode into the artery, with catastrophic and often fatal bleeding.

The major lesion in the thorax is female breast cancer and, less often, large sarcomas that may encompass the abdominal region as well. Perineal ulcerating wounds are frequently seen after the recurrence of a gynecologic cancer. The formation of a fistula is often an associated problem. Rectovaginal, rectovesical, or rectoperineal fistulas are best treated by permanently diverting the fecal stream, such as with an end-colostomy. On the other hand, vesicovaginal or vesicoperineal fistulas are difficult to manage. Procedures to divert urine are usually not practical for these patients because of their short survival. Another complication of perineal ulceration is the presence of a constant bloody ooze.

Abdominal cancers can grow out of stomas and drain sites, causing obstruction, bleeding, and necrosis with malodorous sequelae. A related problem is that of subcutaneous and fascial infections adjacent to ulcerating tumors on the abdominal wall. Finally, large fungating lesions may involve the extremities and, in some instances, require palliative amputation.

MANAGEMENT

The smell of malignant ulceration is due to the presence of anaerobic organisms. These organisms flourish in the accessible necrotic tissues of fungating tumors, and the malodorous volatile fatty acids are released as a metabolic end-product. These fatty acids are responsible for the offensive and penetrating smell (Editorial 1990a). Brusis and Luckhaupt (1989) studied 31 patients with extensive tumors of the head and neck that emitted a putrid odor. Bacteriologic examinations were done either on smears of the ulcerating tumors or on samples of the tumors themselves. Distinct populations of anaerobes were always present. The most frequently demonstrated organism was *Bacteroides melaninogenicus*. This *Bacteroides* species, the authors thought, was responsible for the fetid odor.

Good local care is of utmost importance in managing patients with this problem. Keeping the area of the fungating mass dry and clean often prevents superimposed infections. Wood (1980) suggested cleansing with an inexpensive solution consisting of equal parts of hydrogen peroxide and normal saline. After twice-daily lavage, a small gauze packing soaked in 0.25 percent Dakin solution (sodium hypochlorite) overnight helps to lessen the smell. Daily charcoal dressing, which absorbs the volatile fatty acids, is sometimes sufficient to control the odor (Ashford et al. 1984; Editorial 1990a). Topical honey and icing sugar have also been suggested (Editorial 1990a). This preparation is thought to act by absorption and by the creation of a hyperosmolar environment that prevents bacterial growth. However, the sterility of honey is not assured, and neither agent is practical to use.

Another complication of malignant ulceration is a constant bloody drainage, especially with perineal lesions. Packing the wound with gauze or coagulation material such as absorbable gelatin sponge can sometimes slow this blood loss. In those instances where the mass is large and encompasses a whole region with hemorrhagic potential, the clinician should consider major vessel ligation.

A unique palliative approach of radical surgical debridement for uncontrollable, recurrent pelvic tumors ulcerating through the perineum was described by Temple and Ketcham (1990). Seven patients, with a mean age of 61 years, were treated surgically with tumor resection including a portion of the sacrum to obtain all but the deep margins clear of tumor. Coverage was maintained with myocutaneous flaps. All patients had cancers that had failed to respond to treatment with chemotherapy and radiation. After the surgical debridement, all patients achieved significant relief of pain. Three of the seven patients returned to work, and the remaining four led a relatively comfortable existence at home until death. The median survival of six patients after surgery was 11 months. At the time of the report, one patient was alive at 13 months.

The deodorizing effect of metronidazole was first described in 1980 and then confirmed in 1984. Ashford et al. (1984) performed a prospective double-blind, cross-over trial comparing metronidazole with placebo in nine patients with recurrent breast cancer. For all patients the smell was troublesome. Metronidazole was given for 14 days at a dosage of 200 mg three times daily in the treatment arm of the study. The smell was significantly less after metronidazole than after placebo, as was the difference in anaerobic isolates. According to the authors, the results clearly showed that metronidazole eliminated anaerobes and reduced the smell of fungating tumors. The net effect was an improvement in the quality of life of their patients with malodorous tumors.

In a similar vein, Brusis and Luckhaupt (1989) gave their patients with head and neck tumors either metronidazole or clindamycin to control the smell. Sixteen patients were treated with clindamycin (two 150-mg capsules four times daily) and 15 were treated with metronidazole (one 250-mg tablet five times daily). The odor disappeared more quickly after treatment with clindamycin than after treatment with metronidazole. The smell dissipated some 12 to 36 hours after the start of therapy.

Unfortunately, both clindamycin and metronidazole have drawbacks. Continuous therapy is necessary because the organisms soon regrow when the treatment is stopped. In addition, metronidazole can cause nausea, and long-term use is associated with neuropathy. The avoidance of alcohol that is necessary with metronidazole treatment may be difficult for some patients (Editorial 1990a).

To bypass these problems, some investigators have explored the use of topical metronidazole. Initial trials with dressings soaked in metronidazole injection preparation, although effective for bed sores and diabetic ulcers, were not totally successful in treating odorous tumors because the absorption was poor. Therefore, the metronidazole was incorporated in an 0.8 percent gel formation for use with daily dressings. A trial in 68 hospice patients with smelly tumors showed that it was totally effective in 50 percent, was reasonably effective in another 46 percent, and ineffective in only 3 patients (Newman, Allwood, and Oakes 1989).

Summary

Malignant intestinal obstruction is an uncommon clinical problem (3% incidence in one series) (Baines, Oliver, and Carter 1985) but is difficult to manage. In inoperable cases, the continuous parenteral infusion of antiemetics, anticholinergics, opioids, and octreotide provides a very viable alternative to prolonged NG suctioning and IV fluids. Thirst and dry mouth are relieved by oral fluids, ice chips, and the like. In cases where the obstruction is proximal (i.e., duodenum and proximal jejunum), NG decompression may be necessary to reduce vomiting due to gastric retention. However, a trial of metoclopramide is appropriate if this obstruction is partial and motility is impaired.

Approximately 12 percent of dying cancer patients present with dysphagia, which is generally related to primary tumors in the head and neck, esophagus, or upper stomach and metastases to lymph nodes in the mediastinum. Although most patients with objective evidence of dysphagia have documented local obstruction, other etiologies for this symptom exist, including inadequate oral hygiene and the dysphagia syndrome due to poor neuromuscular coordination. Conservative treatment with diet, attention to oral hygiene, pain control, dexamethasone, and radiation therapy relieves dysphagia in about 60 percent of patients. Intracavitary irradiation, endoscopic laser therapy, or the insertion of self-expanding metallic stents improves swallowing in more than half of patients.

Abnormal muscular function causing weakness seems to be unrelated to the patient's nutritional status, the size of the muscles, or the tumor mass. Presently, no specific treatment is available. Infrequently, paraneoplastic syndromes (for example, the Eaton-Lambert syndrome in patients with small cell lung carcinoma) produce muscular weakness as a remote effect of the cancer. The de novo appearance of muscular cramps is often associated with an underlying neurologic problem.

Although the occurrence of a large fungating tumor in a patient with advanced and uncontrolled cancer is not common (8%), it is very distressing to the patient and family. Good local care, especially keeping the area of the fungating mass dry and clean, is of utmost importance. Rarely, radical surgical debridement is necessary. Systemic drug therapy with metronidazole and clindamycin is effective in alleviating the odor of these tumors by reducing the offending anaerobic flora; however, it is impractical for long-term use. Topical metronidazole, on the other hand, is very effective in controlling the offensive smell.

Chapter 4

Other Problems of Patients with Nonmalignant Diseases

Dementia

Progressive dementia of the Alzheimer type (DAT) is a neurodegenerative disease with no cure. It affects approximately 2 million Americans and is probably the fourth leading cause of death among elderly people. Evidence suggests that the prevalence of DAT may be extremely high among very old people, nearing 50 percent in persons over 85 years of age. The length of survival with DAT is highly variable and may range from 2 to 16 years after the onset of symptoms (Walsh, Welch, and Larson 1990).

The hallmark of dementia is impairment of recent memory, but thought, judgment, perception, language, and functional abilities also deteriorate. Symptoms gradually worsen, and the clinical course is punctuated by acute intervening episodes. Behavioral symptoms include angry outbursts, violence, depression, suspicion, hallucinations, delusions, wandering, and other disturbing problems. The performance of simple tasks such as eating, dressing, and toileting eventually becomes impossible, and ultimately the patient needs long-term institutional care (Brechling and Kuhn 1989). The management of dementia consists of symptomatic treatment of behavioral problems, insomnia, seizures, and intercurrent illnesses.

In view of the similarities of Alzheimer disease and advanced cancer, it is not surprising that the hospice approach has been advocated for patients with dementia. Volicer et al. (1986) reported their experience in applying the hospice approach to 40 patients with advanced DAT in an intermediate care ward that constituted the inpatient component of the Alzheimer's Disease Research Program at the Bedford (Massachusetts) Division of the Boston Geriatric Research, Education, and Clinical Center.

The authors defined five levels of care depending on the optimality of treatment for each individual patient. The highest level (level 1) was aggressive care, including treatment of coexisting medical conditions, transfer to acute care if necessary, and cardiopulmonary resuscitation if needed. The lowest level (level 5) was supportive care only. That care consisted of do-not-resuscitate orders, a decision not to transfer to an acute care unit, denial of work-up and antibiotic treatment of life-threatening infection (pneumonia, urinary tract infection), and the use of oral fluids only for hydration. Patients were assigned to a level of care after a meeting between the multidisciplinary team and family members. Of the 40 patients, none was assigned to level 1, whereas 19 patients (47.5%) were assigned to level 5. Although the environment and inpatient setting were different from conventional hospice care, the authors used similar philosophies and techniques to ensure maximal patient comfort. These included the maximization of quality of life by the use of recreational and occupational therapies, meticulous nursing care, attention to oral hygiene, the use of low doses of morphine if the patient was restless, the use of atropine to decrease pulmonary secretions, and the use of oxygen if the patient was dyspneic. With this approach, the authors believed that patients' suffering was minimized in the terminal stages of advanced DAT.

One of the clinically relevant aspects of Volicer et al.'s (1986) study was their identification and subsequent management of the infectious complications of advanced DAT. Of the 40 patients in the study, 13 died within the first year. An autopsy was performed in 11 cases, with the finding of pneumonia as the cause of death in 7 cases and sepsis resulting from urinary tract infection as the cause of death in 2 cases. Infection, therefore, was the most common cause of death in this population with advanced DAT. The occurrence of pneumonia was often attributed to the aspiration of solids or liquids as a consequence of dysphagia, or difficulty in swallowing.

Sixty-two percent of the patients were not treated with antibiotics if they developed symptoms of pneumonia. The authors thought that the treatment of infection with antibiotics did not necessarily increase patients' comfort. The authors also did not favor empiric antibiotic therapy without a work-up and thought that the patients' comfort was maintained by the frequent use of analgesics and antipyretics. In addition, preliminary data indicated that the hospice approach did not significantly increase the mortality of patients with DAT.

Lynn (1986), in an accompanying editorial, found these clinical situations to be less clear. She suggested that the elderly person with dementia whose strength is being slowly drained by fever and cough should be given antibiotics and restored to his or her previous level of health.

In a follow-up of their 1986 study, Fabiszewski, Volicer, and Volicer (1990) prospectively evaluated episodes of fever in 104 institutionalized patients with DAT to determine the effect of antibiotic treatment on the outcome of fever. Fever was defined as an unanticipated elevation of rectal temperature to 38.9°C or higher or a temperature of 37.7°C or higher that persisted for more than 24 hours. For patients assigned to the antibiotic group, each episode of fever was evaluated using a standardized protocol that consisted of the notation of subjective complaints, assessing functional status, physical examination, and a battery of radiologic and laboratory tests. During those episodes where the source of the fever was clinically apparent, broad-spectrum antibiotic coverage was started on the completion of the diagnostic protocol. In cases where no source of infection was obvious, the patient was monitored and treated with antipyretics and no antibiotics until the culture results were available. For patients in the palliative group, each episode of fever was evaluated identically to that of the antibiotic group with the deletion of the diagnostic tests. These patients were treated symptomatically with antipyretics, analgesics such as morphine when needed, and other therapeutic modalities, including oxygen, oral hydration, pulmonary toilet, and intensive hospice-like nursing care. During the 34-month observation period, 75 patients developed 172 episodes of fever and 29 patients had no fevers. Fever was present more often in patients with advanced disease. Patients with fever treated with antibiotics were compared to patients with fever treated with comfort care only. The incidence of fever was similar for both groups of patients. A survival analysis showed that, for the more severely affected patients, there was no survival difference between the antibiotic and the palliative group; however, among the less severely affected patients, survival was higher for the antibiotic-treated patients. These results, as interpreted by the investigators, indicate that fever is a common occurrence in institutionalized patients with Alzheimer disease and that palliative care is an appropriate treatment option, especially for the more severely impaired patients with DAT.

Difficulty in swallowing is common for patients with advanced dementia as they become bedridden and dependent in all activities of daily living. Enteral tube feedings are frequently used in this situation, but risks and benefits are unclear. To investigate this issue, Finucane, Christmas, and Travis (1999) searched MEDLINE, 1966 through March 1999, to identify data about whether tube feeding of patients with advanced dementia can prevent aspiration pneumonia, prolong survival, reduce the risk of pressure sores or infections, improve function, or provide palliation. They found no data to suggest that tube feeding improves any of these clinically important outcomes. Significant adverse effects of tube feedings included aspiration, obstruction of the feeding tube, and agitation. The authors concluded that the widespread practice of tube feeding for patients with severe dementia should be discouraged on clinical grounds. In a subsequent publication, Gillick (2000) made the point that not only are feeding tubes ineffective in prolonging life, but their use may also necessitate the need for restraints. Finally, Riesenberg (2000) bemoaned the fact that the hospice model of care for patients with advanced DAT, first published in 1986 (Volicer et al. 1986), has yet to gain widespread acceptance.

Motor Neuron Disease

Motor neuron disease is a heterogeneous group of disorders with varying signs and symptoms, all affecting in some manner the anterior horn cells. The most common subset of motor neuron disease in adults is amyotrophic lateral sclerosis (ALS), which affects not only the anterior horn cells but also the corticospinal tracts. The net effect of the ALS lesion is progressive wasting and weakness of those muscles that have lost their nerve supply, in addition to corticospinal tract signs of spasticity and pathologic reflexes in the absence of sensory findings. In most cases of ALS, intellectual function remains intact. Variants of classical ALS include progressive muscular atrophy and progressive bulbar palsy. Atrophy of the spinal muscles presents a clinical picture of limb weakness and wasting with varying degrees of cranial nerve involvement. Progressive bulbar palsy is dominated by weakness and atrophy of cranial nerves of the lower motor neuron type (Williams and Windebank 1991).

The worldwide incidence of ALS is 0.4 to 1.8 per 100,000 people. The incidence of familial ALS is approximately 5 to 10 percent of all ALS. The male to female ratio is 1.0 to 1.6, and the age of onset is between 50 and 60 years (Mitsumoto, Hanson, and Chad 1988).

About one-third of patients with ALS notice the onset of disease because of fine motor impairment affecting activities like sewing or using tools. Another one-third present with leg weakness, while the remaining one-third complain of dysphagia or dysarthria due to involvement of the corticobulbar tract. While the disease characteristically progresses to involve all muscle groups, involvement of the distal muscles is often more severe than involvement of the proximal muscles.

Weakness of bulbar musculature may cause varying degrees of dysarthria and/or dysphagia. The patient's speech may be difficult to interpret because of slowing, tongue weakness, or difficulty in articulation. The patient may have difficulty in initiating swallowing, and saliva may accumulate in the pharynx, leading to episodes of choking. Some patients may have a hyperactive cough reflex, whereas others may not be able to cough adequately, thus predisposing them to aspiration pneumonia.

The control of bladder, bowel, and autonomic function is generally unimpaired, even late in the disease. Another important feature of ALS is the surprising absence of pressure sores, even in patients bedridden for long periods (Mitsumoto, Hanson, and Chad 1988).

Because of the poor prognosis associated with ALS, it is important for the clinician to confirm the clinical diagnosis by investigative procedures. Among the studies most essential is the electromyogram (EMG), which shows characteristic changes consistent with the diagnosis of ALS. Furthermore, the EMG may be useful in the early stages by establishing the widespread nature of the involvement. Occasionally, computed tomographic (CT) scanning of the spine and magnetic resonance imaging (MRI) are necessary to eliminate other diagnoses, such as degenerative disease of the spine with nerve compression, which can mimic ALS.

The clinical outlook for ALS is bleak, with an average survival of three years. One-half of the patients die in less than three years, with only 20 percent and 10 percent surviving more than 5 and 10 years, respectively. Younger patients with a longer duration before diagnosis and milder involvement at diagnosis have a better prognosis, whereas older patients with a shorter duration and more severe involvement at diagnosis have a poorer prognosis (Mitsumoto, Hanson, and Chad 1988).

Despite ongoing active clinical research, the etiology of ALS remains obscure. Likewise, all therapeutic interventions have been uniformly ineffective. Thus, the major care for patients with ALS remains supportive, not curative.

In an attempt to better understand the problems of caring for patients with ALS and other motor neuron disease at St. Christopher's Hospice in London, Saunders, Walsh, and Smith (1981) retrospectively reviewed their experience with 100 patients. Forty men and 60 women were included in this survey. The median ages were 57 years for men and 64 years for women. The median stay in hospice for men was 80 days, with a wide range from 8 hours to four and one-half years. The women's stay in hospice was shorter, with a median of 32.5 days and a range of 11 hours to 157 weeks. Sixty percent of the patients had noted the onset of the disease between one and three years before admission. In the whole group, paralysis was generally widespread and communication was often difficult.

These patients had a wide range of symptoms. Common symptoms included constipation, dysarthria, dysphagia and choking attacks, dyspnea, insomnia, pain, salivation and secretions, and tiredness. Diarrhea was occasionally a problem, whereas pressure sores, hunger and thirst, and urinary problems were uncommon. The pharmacologic management of these troublesome clinical problems varied by symptoms, but often one drug was used in several different clinical situations. For example, opioids were employed in 84 percent of the patients for pain, dyspnea, misery, anxiety, insomnia, hunger, and thirst. Diazepam was given to 63 percent of the patients to control muscle fasciculations, spasticity, cramps, and anxiety. Finally, tricyclic antidepressants were used in 40 percent of the patients for depression, sadness, and insomnia.

As advocated by Saunders, Walsh, and Smith (1981), the skilled use of small doses of opioids can have a positive effect on the management of this disease. These drugs can be given as effective tranquilizers and hypnotics at an early stage of the disease. During their review, Saunders, Walsh, and Smith (1981) found that the maximal dose of parenteral diamorphine for most patients ranged between 2.5 and 5.0 mg.

A definition of pain was sought from 45 patients, with approximately half complaining of the combination of stiffness, aching, cramping, and burning discomfort. This symptom complex was often well controlled by the use of physiotherapy and by the nonsteroidal anti-inflammatory drugs early and by opioid drugs later.

Parenteral diamorphine combined with chlorpromazine, diazepam, and/or anticholinergics was used for terminal distress of any kind. One or more injections were given in 75 percent of the patients. Of the 100 patients, 94 had died, only 1 in a choking attack.

Death was quick in the majority of cases. The most common clinical picture was of sudden rapid deterioration, frequently starting with an upper respiratory infection and followed by increasing exhaustion and dyspnea. Of the 10 autopsy examinations done, 6 showed widespread bronchial pneumonia.

Finally, the patients' moods ranged from depressed to anxious/frightened. Saunders, Walsh, and Smith (1981) thought that their emotional liability was a little greater than would be expected of a normal person with limited communication ability. The authors also emphasized the importance of distinguishing sadness and frustration from a true depressive reaction. Of the 15 patients admitted to hospice on tricyclic antidepressants, only 4 were considered to be depressed on admission. On the other hand, 14 patients who were considered to be depressed were not receiving antidepressants. Some 40 percent of patients were treated with tricyclic antidepressants, not only for depression but also for sedation and the anticholinergic beneficial side effect. Only 14 percent of the patients were referred for psychiatric consultation. The investigators thought that dying of ALS was no more a psychiatric problem in itself than was dying of cancer.

In an updated review of the St. Christopher's experience, O'Brien, Kelly, and Saunders (1992) highlighted the response of symptom control to opioid treatment in 124 patients with motor neuron disease. Of the 57 percent of patients with pain, three-quarters obtained good pain control with opioids. Dyspnea, occurring in 47 percent of the patients, also responded favorably to the use of opioids in 81 percent of the cases. Insomnia, likewise, was well controlled with opioids in the great majority (82%) of patients with this problem (48%). The mean dosage of opioid (oral morphine equivalent) was 30 mg/24 hours and the mean duration of the treatment was 58 days. Many patients were noted to deteriorate suddenly, and in 58 percent of the cases death occurred within 24 hours of this deterioration. When dying, 106 patients (94%) were peaceful and relaxed; 101 patients (89%) received opioids during this dying period. No patient choked to death. In fact, the authors strenuously objected to the term *choking* and thought it is both inappropriate and inaccurate in describing the cause of death in motor neuron disease; they advocated the abandonment of its use.

Acquired Immunodeficiency Syndrome (AIDS)

Since the initial description of AIDS in 1981, more than 550,000 cases of AIDS have been reported in the United States and more than half (60%) of these patients have died. The Centers for Disease Control (CDC) estimated that there were approximately 750,000 HIV-infected individuals in the United States at the beginning of 1986, and by the late 1990s, 1 million people were infected with HIV (Ferri 1998).

Initially, AIDS was a disease of homosexual and bisexual men. In the United States, the proportion of persons with AIDS who are homosexual has fallen, while the proportion of men or women with AIDS whose risk behavior is heterosexual has increased. The proportion of intravenous drug users with AIDS has remained stable. Adolescent women are the fastest-growing group of those newly diagnosed with AIDS. Seventy percent of women with AIDS either are intravenous drug users or are heterosexual partners of intravenous drug users. Worldwide, women who acquire HIV through heterosexual contact comprise the greatest proportion of cases of AIDS (Ferri 1998). The incidence of new cases of AIDS acquired by blood transfusion and replacement of clotting factor has stabilized as a result of screening blood and blood products (Gold 1992). The number of cases in infants born to HIV-infected women has increased to 2,000 per year.

Patients with AIDS have a wide variety of opportunistic infections and malignant neoplasms (Kaplan, Wofsy, and Volberding 1987). Of all the opportunistic infections, *Pneumocystis carinii* pneumonia is the most common. Patients generally present with fever, nonproductive cough, and exertional shortness of breath. Symptoms of cryptococcal meningitis include a high fever and headache. Toxoplasmosis is a common cause of central nervous system disease in patients with AIDS. Focal neurologic findings, seizures, fever, or a decreased level of consciousness is often found. *Cryptosporidium* is frequently associated with severe and chronic watery diarrhea, which can lead to dehydration and wasting. Both *Mycobacterium avium* and *Mycobacterium tuberculosis* infections are frequently seen in patients with AIDS. Oropharyngitis due to candidal infection is the most common fungal infection encountered. It is present in the majority of patients with AIDS at some time during the course of the disease. Infections of herpes simplex virus are common and may be severe and persistent.

Cytomegalovirus (CMV) is a frequent cause of morbidity and mortality. CMV is often associated with pneumonitis, retinitis, cerebritis, or colitis.

Like the opportunistic infections, malignant neoplasms associated with AIDS (namely, Kaposi sarcoma and non-Hodgkin lymphoma) are difficult to treat. Since most patients with AIDS die of opportunistic infections rather than Kaposi sarcoma, treatment is aimed at reducing the morbidity of advanced Kaposi sarcoma, such as the bulky, painful skin or oropharyngeal lesions. Since neither antibiotic therapy for opportunistic infections nor chemotherapy and radiation therapy for malignant neoplasms is able to reverse the underlying immune defect in AIDS, new forms of treatment were developed specifically to have an impact on this immunodeficiency state. One such treatment is the antiviral agent azidothymidine (AZT), or Zidovudine. As reported preliminarily by Yarchoan and Broder (1987), the drug was given for up to 18 months to AIDS patients. The results showed an improvement in immunologic function, a reversal (at least partially) in neurologic dysfunction for some patients, and an improvement in certain other clinical AIDS-associated abnormalities. The average survival of 10 months that was originally reported in these patients has now been extended to approximately two years with the use of AZT (Redfield and Tramont 1989). AZT given to asymptomatic patients and to patients with AIDS-related complex (ARC) delays the onset of AIDS; however, the benefits of AZT therapy are not permanent, and AIDS will develop in most HIV-infected patients (Gold 1992). More recently, using combination antiretroviral therapy in triple drug regimens has resulted in declines in morbidity and mortality among patients with human immunodeficiency virus (Ferri 1998).

Patients with advanced or terminal stages of AIDS share many of the same symptoms of patients dying of other diseases, such as cancer. Chronic infections and skin problems, however, are uniquely found in the patient dying with AIDS. Moss (1991) retrospectively reviewed the first 100 consecutive admissions to a new palliative care unit for AIDS patients. The vast majority of the patients were men who had contracted the disease by homosexual contact or intravenous drug use. The ages ranged from 20 to 70 years, with 78 percent being between 30 and 49 years. All of these patients had a number of coexisting diagnoses, usually three or four, and most of these were opportunistic infections for which active treatment, maintenance therapy, or prophylaxis was being given. For example, 68 percent of the patients had prior candidal infection, and 64 percent of these were receiving active therapy or prophylaxis. More than half (59%) had had one or more previous episodes of *P. carinii* pneumonia, and 60 percent of these patients were taking prophylactic drugs. The 18 patients (22%) with a diagnosis of mycobacterial disease were taking several antituberculous drugs, and 22 (28%) had a diagnosis of cytomegalovirus retinitis. As a result of these coexisting problems, polypharmacy was inevitable. A total of 48 percent of the patients were taking 4 to 6 drugs, and 30 percent were taking 7 to 10 drugs. About one-third of the patients were receiving AZT and continued to do so until the very end.

Pain was a frequently (84%) encountered symptom. Pain due to HIV-related demyelinating peripheral neuropathy was the most common (22%), followed by pain from pressure sores, visceral pain, total body pain, headache, joint pain, epigastric/retrosternal pain, muscle pain, and anorectal discomfort. Unlike the causes of pain in dying cancer patients, some sources of discomfort in AIDS patients were related to infections and drugs. For example, headaches were often associated with infection of the central nervous system, such as cryptococcal meningitis or cerebral toxoplasmosis. Retrosternal or epigastric pain usually was related to the presence of candidal esophagitis. Finally, myopathic pain correlated with the use of AZT, especially in high doses.

Other common symptoms noted by Moss (1991) were weight loss, anorexia, confusion, nausea and vomiting, depression, cough, diarrhea, constipation, dyspnea, and paralysis (table 4.1). Skin problems were extremely common (45%). About 20 percent of the patients had dry skin, which predisposed to bacterial skin infections. Tinea and other fungal infections were frequent. Fourteen percent of the patients had seborrheic dermatitis, which was often linked to fungal infections. Scabies infection was noted in 7 percent of the patients.

Psychiatric problems, such as anxiety and depression, are common with AIDS patients but must be distinguished from AIDS-related dementia, which occurs in at least half of the patients before death. HIV has been shown to have direct effects on the central nervous system; nevertheless, most HIV-infected asymptomatic patients evidence no clinically significant mental changes. A few, however, show a subtle dementia characterized by apathy, social withdrawal, the avoidance of complex tasks, and mental slowing. As death approaches, more significant dementia develops, but at this point it is difficult to discern the degree to which the cognitive decline is due to the direct effects of HIV on the central nervous

TABLE 4.1   Common Symptoms of 100
Patients with Advanced AIDS

Symptom (%)	Frequency
Pain	84
Weight loss	61
Skin problems	45
Anorexia	41
Confusion	29
Nausea and vomiting	21
Depression	20
Cough	19
Diarrhea	18
Constipation	18
Dyspnea	11
Paralysis	8

Source: Moss (1991).

system, systemic illness, infection, tumor, or the effects of various medications (Jacobsberg and Perry 1992).

The control of pain and symptoms for terminally ill patients with AIDS is similar to that outlined for other diseases, such as cancer. Indeed, megestrol acetate has shown a salutary effect on appetite and weight gain in AIDS patients with anorexia and cachexia (Von Roenn, Murphy, and Wegener 1990). No randomized clinical trial on the use of corticosteroids in patients with advanced AIDS has been reported, although Cole (1991) advocated their generalized use based on his personal experience.

Because of the known polypharmacy (Wood, Whittet, and Bradbeer 1997) in AIDS patients, clinicians must consider stopping as many medications as possible to avoid undue toxicity and potential drug interactions. The treatment of candidiasis and prophylaxis against herpes simplex reactivation should be continued as long as possible, since the morbidity of these conditions is high and their progression does not cause a rapid demise. Although the treatment of mycobacterial disease occasionally produces a beneficial effect, it can be discontinued and fever and sweating can be controlled with antipyretic drugs.

It is also reasonable to stop parenteral therapy for cytomegalovirus retinitis, since more than half of patients do not develop progressive retinitis until after three weeks after drug discontinuation or beyond. Since the benefit of AZT in advanced AIDS has not been established, this drug should also be stopped, with patient concurrence. Medications for pain and symptoms, such as acetaminophen, morphine, and nonsteroidal anti-inflammatories, compete with AZT for hepatic metabolism and can increase serum levels of AZT to potentially toxic heights. Finally, Cole (1991) did not personally observe reactivation or symptomatic progression of opportunistic infections after stopping treatment.

Anecdotal case reports have, on occasion, demonstrated that the transmission of HIV to a health care worker can result from various modes of exposure to HIV, such as contaminated hollow-bore needles with parenteral injury, cuts, mucosal splashes, or skin contact. Some cases of HIV transmission related to needlestick injury involved only limited blood infusion or a relatively superficial injury. Epidemiologic studies of occupational risks of transmission have shown that persons who have had parenteral exposure have the greatest risk (i.e., about 0.5%). The observed risk associated with known exposure via mucosal membrane and skin is close to 0 (Weiss 1992; Ferri 1998).

Chronic Vegetative State

The care of terminally ill patients, especially those in a chronic vegetative state, can be very trying. Because of this, Carlson, Devich, and Frank (1988) developed a comprehensive support care team in a major teaching hospital to manage these patients. The team included a physician and a clinical nurse specialist who provided primary medical care, family support, and in-service guidance to the hospital staff about ethical issues. Nursing, pastoral care, social work, and other hospital services were incorporated into a multidisciplinary approach.

The goals of the comprehensive support care team were:

- to provide a hospital service dedicated to consistent and humane care of the hopelessly ill patient and support of their families;
- to develop a treatment plan for each patient that reflected ethical decision making involving the patient and proxy/family;
- to provide comprehensive but conservative care using a multidisciplinary approach;
- to facilitate access to institutional and community support services;
- to promote learning about and discussion of ethical issues by the hospital staff.

During an 18-month period, 212 patients were accepted on the team's service. The mean age of the patients was 67 years, with a range of 17 to 100 years. The most common diagnosis was global central nervous system anoxia following cardiopulmonary arrest in 62 patients (29%). A variety of other neurologic disorders accounted for 79 patients (37%). Therefore, for 141 patients (67%) under the team's care, dysfunction of the central nervous system was a major clinical feature. Diagnoses in the remaining patients included cancer (16%), gastrointestinal (predominantly hepatic) failure (7%), renal failure (4%), pulmonary failure (2%), metabolic abnormalities (2%), cardiovascular problems (1%), and AIDS (1%). Most patients (78%) were receiving mechanical ventilation when accepted on the service. About one-third of these patients were weaned from assisted ventilation. An additional 17 percent were terminally weaned with discontinuation of ventilatory life support. The mean length of the hospital stay was 26 days for all patients, with a mean length of stay under the care of this team of 9 days. Only 6 patients (3%), all comatose, were discharged home; another 25 patients (12%) were transferred to an extended care facility. The remaining patients either died (82%) or were returned to their primary care service (3%). Survival rates were very similar when comparing before, early, and late management by the team in patients with global anoxic brain injury. However, there was a progressive decrease in the length of stay in the hospital corresponding to the full development of the team service. It was the authors' hope that this approach to the care of terminally ill patients, especially those in coma, would serve as an alternative method of treatment in similar hospital settings.

Advanced Pulmonary Disease

Advanced pulmonary disease, usually due to chronic bronchitis or emphysema, is very similar to advanced cancer in that it is progressive, is incurable, and causes distressing symptoms, ultimately leading to death (Kinzel 1991). The treatment of the symptoms of patients with advanced pulmonary disease is the same as that previously described for other terminal diseases except in the management of hypoxia, infections, dyspnea, and panic attacks.

Hypoxia is present in the majority of symptomatic patients with advanced pulmonary disease. The hemoglobin oxygen saturation should be maintained above 90 percent, with supplemental oxygen to maintain the function of the cardiovascular and central nervous systems.

Recurrent pulmonary infections are common in advanced pulmonary disease and frequently are the cause of death. When death is not imminent, treating the pulmonary infection is essential in relieving dyspnea. Treatment is usually empiric. Broad-spectrum antibiotics should be started when shortness of breath worsens and is associated with a change in sputum or when other signs of infection are present.

Dyspnea is the cardinal symptom of patients with advanced pulmonary disease. It may be caused by hypoxia, congestive heart failure, tenacious secretions, minor infections, ischemic heart disease, pleural effusion, reflux esophagitis, or emotional distress. Because there is no uniformly effective method of alleviating dyspnea, the clinician should search for and appropriately manage any complicating medical conditions, such as congestive heart failure. Pulmonary function should be optimized by good pulmonary toilet, theophylline, inhaled or oral beta agonists, inhaled atropine derivatives, steroids, and low-flow oxygen. Theophylline can be given effectively orally with a once-daily preparation, usually given at bedtime. The blood levels of theophylline need to be monitored periodically to minimize toxicity. Beta agonists, mainly albuterol or metaproteranol, are administered by a hand-held multidose inhaler, usually with a spacer device. Two inhalations four times daily is the standard dosage; however, in very late stage patients who benefit from inhaled beta agonists, doses may be increased to three inhalations every four hours. Ipratropium (an atropine derivative) may also be helpful when used as two inhalations four times daily. Finally, morphine in doses of 2.5 to 10 mg orally every four to six hours is useful in relieving dyspnea.

Panic is the most dramatic emotional symptom of patients with advanced pulmonary disease. It is associated with a rapid exacerbation of symptoms into a vicious cycle: panic causing increased bronchospasm, leading to increasing dyspnea, leading to further panic. Strong emotional support, along with an increase in the inhaled beta agonist, may relieve minor attacks. Treatment with 0.25 mg subcutaneous terbutaline or 3 to 5 mg subcutaneous morphine is more effective (Kinzel 1991).

Heart Disease

Congestive heart failure is the only major cardiovascular disease with increasing incidence, prevalence, and mortality. A study of 20 English health districts investigated symptoms of patients dying of heart failure. Patients who died from heart disease, including heart failure, experienced a wide range of symptoms, often distressing and lasting more than six months. Dyspnea, pain, nausea, constipation, and low mood were common and poorly controlled. At least one in six symptoms was as severe as those of patients with cancer managed in hospices or by palliative care services (Gibbs, Addington-Hall, and Gibbs 1998).

As noted by O'Brien, Welsh, and Dunn (1998), certain clinical aspects of heart failure are similar to those of cancer. For example, both types of patients may have dyspnea, lethargy, anorexia and cachexia, nausea, constipation, poor mobility, depression, cough, dizziness or postural hypotension, jaundice, and polypharmacy. In contrast with cancer patients,

patients with terminal heart failure have more edema, and predicting their life expectancy is not as accurate.

Standard treatment with diuretics, digoxin, and angiotensin-converting enzyme (ACE) inhibitors should be continued, since these treatment modalities have been shown to improve symptoms (Brozena 1999). Some patients, however, may not tolerate the blood pressure–lowering effects of ACE inhibitors, which should be stopped in such cases.

Increased doses of diuretics, often given intravenously, may be needed to treat the dyspnea, orthopnea, edema, and at times ascites that accompany end-stage heart failure. Potassium and magnesium supplements may be needed to avoid muscle cramps that may be precipitated by electrolyte deficiency. Other methods of treatment of dyspnea include oxygen and nitrates. Sublingual nitroglycerine is especially helpful in the management of paroxysmal episodes. Oral morphine can be used to control breathlessness, and, for selected patients, a morphine infusion can be used to treat more severe dyspnea. Thoracentesis and/or paracentesis are usually reserved for cases in which the clinician has a particular reason to believe that these procedures may improve their patients' symptoms. For selected patients, intravenous inotropic agents may be an option if the above measures fail to control symptoms (Brozena 1999).

Finally, it is important for the clinician to recognize that patients with heart failure are more likely to die suddenly than are patients with cancer, and they do not necessarily have a clearly defined terminal phase (Gibbs, Addington-Hall, and Gibbs 1998).

Summary

Progressive dementia of the Alzheimer type has no cure. Like advanced cancer, it follows a relentless downhill clinical course punctuated by acute intervening episodes, predominantly infectious in nature. For severely impaired patients, the management of the symptoms of these episodes (generally pneumonia) with antipyretics, analgesics, and intensive nursing care produces the same outcome as does more aggressive treatment using diagnostic tests and antibiotics. Tube feeding is harmful rather than beneficial for these patients.

Likewise, there is no curative therapy for motor neuron diseases such as ALS; there is only supportive care. Common symptoms include dysarthria, dysphagia, choking attacks, dyspnea, constipation, insomnia, pain, salivation, excessive secretions, and tiredness. Small doses of opioids are extremely effective in managing not only pain but also other symptoms.

Patients with AIDS encounter many of the same problems as patients dying of other diseases. Chronic infections and skin disorders, however, are uniquely found in the patient dying of AIDS. Pain is the most frequent symptom and is often due to HIV-related demyelinating peripheral neuropathy. The control of pain and other symptoms in these patients is very similar to that outlined for other diseases, including the use of megestrol acetate for anorexia and cachexia. Avoid polypharmacy to prevent undue toxicity and drug interactions.

The use of a comprehensive support care team to manage the comatose patient in a chronic vegetative state is an enlightened approach to a most difficult problem.

The treatment of the symptoms of patients with advanced pulmonary disease differs from that of other terminal illnesses in the management of hypoxia, infections, dyspnea, and panic attacks. The clinician should use supplemental oxygen for hypoxia, and administer antibiotics for pulmonary infections; to lessen dyspnea and optimize pulmonary function by good pulmonary toilet and the use of theophylline, beta agonists, atropine derivatives, steroids, low-flow oxygen, and low doses of morphine; and manage panic attacks with strong emotional support, inhaled beta agonists, terbutaline, or small doses of morphine.

Heart failure shares many of the same clinical problems evident in cancer patients. Unlike patients with cancer, however, patients with heart failure are more prone to sudden death and generally do not have a clearly defined terminal phase. Treatment includes diuretics, digoxin, oxygen, sublingual nitroclycerine, and, in some instances, inotropic agents. Dyspnea is managed with morphine and thoracentesis and/or paracentesis when necessary.

Chapter 5

Palliative Surgery

Although surgical intervention is infrequent in dying patients, palliative surgery plays an important role, much like chemotherapy and radiation therapy, in the management of these patients' symptoms. As noted by Forbes (1988), the overall goal of palliative surgery is to improve the patient's quality of life by appropriately reducing symptoms without undue surgical complication. To this end, Forbes reviewed the basic principles relevant to the surgical management of patients with advanced cancer (table 5.1):

- Patients with cancer undergoing surgery are primarily surgical patients. Therefore, it is important to address the physical and psychological stresses generally associated with any surgical procedure.
- Surgery is directed at the consequences of the tumor. Morbidity in advanced cancer often results from the anatomic location of the tumor. For example, advanced head and neck cancers have the potential to erode the carotid artery, resulting in dramatic and explosive bleeding. Palliative surgery can prevent this event. Hence, surgical intervention in patients with advanced cancer should be aimed at the symptoms rather than at the overall malignant process.
- Integrate surgery into both specific treatment and supportive care programs. Surgery for palliation must be an integral part of the patient's total management plan.
- Avoid unreasonably delaying palliative surgery. The patient's quality of life is best improved by quickly relieving the distressful symptoms and by avoiding the anxiety associated with the uncertainty of future management plans.
- Surgical problems may have a benign cause; obtain histologic findings where possible. The following examples of definitive palliative surgery illustrate the uncertain intent of surgery before the procedure. Patients with obstructive jaundice and known cancer may have liver metastases, extrahepatic biliary obstruction due to lymph node metastases, or a benign etiology such as cholelithiasis. In this case,

TABLE 5.1   An Overview of Palliative Surgery

The role of surgery in palliation:
    Cancer patients are surgical patients first.
    Surgery is directed at the consequences of the tumor.
    Integrate surgery into both specific treatment and supportive care programs.
    Avoid unreasonable delay of palliative surgery.
    Surgical problems may have a benign cause; obtain histologic findings where possible.
Principles of preoperative care:
    Consultations and explanations.
    Planning for immediate and long-term care.
Principles of operating for advanced cancer:
    Determining site of incision.
    Each patient must undergo the procedure that is optimal for him or her.
Principles of postoperative care:
    Optimize recovery by avoiding complications.
    Early diagnosis and aggressive management of complications.

Source: Forbes (1988).

surgical exploration will establish the etiology of jaundice and, if feasible, appropriate surgery can be performed. Intestinal obstruction
may well be due to recurrent or progressive disease in patients with
known ovarian or colorectal cancer. However, in one-third of the
cases, the obstruction will be caused by a benign process such as adhesions, internal hernias, or radiation enteritis.

Principles of Preoperative Care

- The clinician must carefully explain to the patient and family the bur-
  dens and benefits of the planned surgery. Likewise, he or she should
  fully discuss anticipated outcomes without surgical intervention.
- Preoperative planning for immediate and long-term care is essential.
  The results of palliative surgery may depend largely on the adequacy
  of the preoperative preparation and assessment. Cancer patients can
  experience all the major complications of surgery during and after
  operations and, depending on their overall medical status, may have
  these complications more frequently and to a more severe degree.
  Thus, preoperative evaluation should include not only the tumor
  type and stage of disease but also the general medical status of the
  patient.
    The postoperative recovery environment and length of time
  should be clearly established before the procedure is undertaken. If
  the patient is likely to have a long recovery period with only a short

hospitalization with intensive nursing, then appropriate plans must be made for care in the home or another outpatient setting.

Principles of Operating for Advanced Cancer

- The site of the incision is crucial. A poorly placed incision can compromise an otherwise successful operation. Incisions in patients with advanced cancer may heal slowly. Incisions should be placed where they provide good access and healing. Some incision sites, such as the lower midline abdomen, are notoriously poor at healing and should be avoided. In a similar fashion, prior areas of radiation therapy are not desirable sites for incision.
- Each patient must undergo the procedure that is optimal for him or her. The surgery is tailored to each patient's individual needs and medical status. For example, the decision to attempt a resection or bypass procedure for bowel obstruction depends on the patient's fitness and age and the available postoperative care facilities. A noncurative resection of bowel obstruction with an anastomosis and tumor removal might well be a better palliative procedure in terms of quality of life than a simple short bypass that is likely to cause additional complications or continued pain due to the presence of a tumor. The decision as to whether or not to resect bowel may be complicated by prior radiation therapy.

Principles of Postoperative Care

- Optimize the recovery by avoiding complications. Postoperative complications can be avoided or minimized by good preoperative planning, especially by assuring that optimal postoperative care is available. Many patients with cancer have an impaired nutritional status, and every attempt should be made to address and correct this, if possible, before surgery.
- Early diagnosis and aggressive management of complications are important. All surgical complications can be particularly troublesome in cancer patients; these include bleeding, infection, poor wound healing, electrolyte and acid-base disorders, renal failure, airway obstruction, and problems related to prolonged immobilization (such as pressure sores, pulmonary embolus, muscle wasting, and psychological stress from inactivity and prolonged hospitalization). Many of these complications are potentially fatal and therefore should be treated early and aggressively.

There are a paucity of scientific data and controlled clinical trials to determine the proper role of palliative surgery for advanced cancer. Surgical interventions are consequently based largely on principles, experience, and information from surgery in other settings, and new scientific investigations are required.

Indications for Surgery

As noted by Veronisi (1982), the indications for palliative surgery are less well defined than are those for curative surgery, and they must be weighed on an individual basis in the light of the rate of disease progression, the life expectancy, the seriousness of the disturbance produced by the disease, and the degree of improvement of symptoms that can be expected. As a general rule, palliative surgery is contemplated for lesions causing obstruction, compression, bleeding, pain, and other symptoms.

OBSTRUCTION

Surgical intervention for obstruction is usually directed at the gastrointestinal tract, the genitourinary tract, the bile ducts, and the blood vessels. Patients with obstructions of the respiratory tract or lymphatic system rarely need surgery.

Obstructions of the gastrointestinal tract are the ones that most often require surgical intervention. The most frequent sites are the esophagus, the gastric pylorus, the small bowel, and the distal large bowel. Patency of the esophagus can be maintained by the insertion of an intracavitary prosthesis, and pyloric obstruction can be managed by creating a gastroenteric anastomosis. When feasible, bowel obstruction is dealt with by resection, bypass, or, in the case of large bowel tumors, colostomy. An obstruction of the ureter is not uncommon with pelvic tumors and may occur either unilaterally or bilaterally. The ureters can be given an outlet either on the skin or into the large intestine. Also, a nephrostomy can be performed. Lower urinary tract obstruction can be managed by using a cystostomy.

In recent years, several studies have been published showing the safety and efficacy of expandable metal stents for the relief of symptoms in patients with inoperable colorectal cancer causing obstruction. Muir (1999) reviewed these studies and reported that the symptoms of obstruction were effectively relieved in 48 to 72 hours in over 90 percent of the cases, with fairly low rates of complication. The most common complications were pain (10–15%) due to stent placement and bleeding (8–12%). There was one case of intestinal perforation and several cases of stent migration after placement (8–36%); stent occlusion, usually due to tumor progression, was infrequent (4–18%). Mean survival of patients after stent placement was 5.7 months, which is comparable to that of patients who received surgical intervention, but without the risk of operative morbidity and mortality. As noted by Muir (1999), there have been no studies randomizing these two interventions and there are no data comparing outcomes of conservative medical management to outcomes of stent placement. Finally, both surgical intervention and stent placement are problematic for patients with multiple sites of obstruction.

Tumors causing obstruction of a bile duct are usually cancers of the head of the pancreas or, more rarely, metastatic lymph nodes of the porta hepatis. In these instances, good palliation can be achieved by diversion of the bile flow into the jejunum or stomach.

Finally, operations for arterial occlusion are rare but may be necessary, as in the case of occlusion of the common carotid artery by metastases from head and neck cancers.

COMPRESSION OF THE SPINAL CORD

Approximately half of the patients with compression of the spinal cord have advanced disease with metastases (Forbes 1988). The early diagnosis of this problem is important to prevent the tragedy of a patient with permanent paraplegia. Although opinions differ as to the exact role and timing of surgery (decompressive laminectomy) and radiation therapy, procrastination is to be avoided. Husband (1998) investigated the delay in presentation, diagnosis, and treatment of malignant spinal cord compression in 301 consecutive patients at a regional cancer center. The median delay from the onset of symptoms of cord compression to treatment was 14 days, with a range of 0 to 840 days. In general, cord compression should be diagnosed and treated within 24 hours for optimal functional outcome. Husband (1998) found that this target was not achieved for 70 percent of patients at the family practitioner stage, 79 percent at the general hospital stage, and 33 percent at the treatment unit stage. The author concluded that the failure to diagnose spinal cord compression and the failure to investigate, refer, and treat with sufficient urgency were the main causes of delay and the consequent deterioration in function.

Sorensen et al. (1990), in a seven-year retrospective review, studied the outcome of 345 patients treated for metastatic spinal cord compression with radiation therapy alone, laminectomy alone, or laminectomy followed by radiation therapy. Carcinomas of the lung, prostate, breast, and kidney were the most common malignancies causing cord compression. The outcome of therapy depended primarily on the patient's ambulatory status at the time of the diagnosis. The majority of the patients (79%) who

were able to walk before treatment remained ambulatory, in contrast to
the 21 percent of the nonambulatory paraplegic patients and the 6 percent of the paralytic patients who regained the ability to walk. Patients
managed with laminectomy followed by radiation therapy responded better than did patients treated with radiation therapy or laminectomy
alone; when the patient's pretreatment motor status was considered, however, there was no significant difference among the three forms of therapy. In the subgroup of nonambulatory patients, however, a significantly
better restoration of gait was observed in patients treated with combined
laminectomy and radiation therapy than in patients treated with radiation therapy alone. The median survival of all patients was 3.1 months.
The results of this study, as suggested by the investigators, point out the
need for a prospective, randomized study to answer the question as to
which modality or combination is optimal for the treatment of metastatic compression of the spinal cord.

BLEEDING

Although it would be distinctly unusual, surgery can play a vital role in
the management of bleeding problems. Bleeding from gastric infiltration
from advanced lymphoma or carcinoma may require gastric resection if
nonsurgical measures are not successful (Veronisi 1982). As noted previously, explosive bleeding from tumor erosion into the carotid artery may
require surgical intervention.

PAIN

Neurosurgical procedures can play an important part in managing
pain. This will be discussed in part II.

FRACTURE

Surgery is indicated for patients with metastatic bone disease causing
pathologic fractures and pain. The aims of this orthopedic intervention
are to control pain and preserve remaining function so patients can be
mobilized.

Bono et al. (1991) reported the results of palliative surgery for metastatic bone disease performed during a 10-year period. Among 349 patients
with bone metastases, 83 (24%) required one or more surgical procedures. The most common tumor sites were breast, lung, prostate, and kidney. A variety of orthopedic procedures were employed. Of the total of
83 patients with metastatic bone disease, surgery was done in 19 patients
at the prefracture stage, in 54 patients after complete fracture, and in 10

patients to decompress the spinal cord. Positive short-term results were obtained for more than 75 percent of the patients, with a mean survival time of 11.4 months. Seven patients developed mild complications. The clinician should consider surgical intervention if metastatic bone pain is not relieved by other means; if fracture is imminent, as indicated by the loss of more than half the cortical bone thickness, or if a fracture has already occurred (Editorial 1992).

OTHER SYMPTOMS

Dramatic as it sounds, amputation is occasionally a useful operation for patients with advanced cancer. Specifically, it is indicated in peripheral solid and bone tumors that are unresponsive to radiation therapy and are painful, are in danger of fungation, or grossly interfere with function by virtue of bulk (Philips 1984).

Patients requiring multiple paracenteses for recurrent malignant ascites may be candidates for the placement of a peritoneovenous shunt (LeVeen or Denver shunt). Although the concept of returning ascitic fluid to the intravascular space is not new, improvement in technology with peritoneovenous devices has led to their widespread use. These devices consist of a length of multiply perforated tube inserted in the peritoneal cavity, a length of tubing placed into the superior vena cava or right atrium, and a unidirectional flow valve connecting the two arms (Baker 1989). The main difference between the LeVeen and Denver shunts is the one-way valve in the Denver shunt that can be manually pumped to flush any accumulated debris at periodic intervals. Despite this theoretical advantage of the Denver shunt, clinically there is no difference in effectiveness of the two shunts.

Baker (1989) summarized the results of 15 reported studies involving 372 patients managed by the placement of a peritoneovenous shunt to control malignant ascites. The majority of patients had ovarian, gastrointestinal, or breast cancer. The median survivals ranged from 5 to 16 weeks, with 0 to 12 percent alive at one year. Response to shunting varied from 32 to 100 percent, with most studies reporting good to excellent relief of symptoms.

Summary

Palliative surgery, much like other modalities of controlling pain and symptoms, plays an important role in the medical management of dying patients. Basic principles relevant to surgery have been delineated (see table 5.1). Indications are less well defined for palliative surgery than for curative surgery, and must be individualized. In general, the clinician should contemplate palliative surgery for lesions causing obstruction, compression of the spinal cord, bleeding, pain (see part II), fracture, and other symptoms. Prospective clinical trials are needed to define clearly the role of palliative surgery for patients with advanced cancer.

The Management of Pain

Chapter 6

An Overview of Pain Management

Recent publicity regarding euthanasia (Humphry 1991; Enck 1999) has clearly focused for the medical community the issue of pain control in the dying patient. Existing information suggests that one-third of cancer patients undergoing active treatment and 60 to 90 percent of patients with advanced disease experience moderate to severe pain (Foley 1985). In addition, some 20 to 50 percent of patients with all stages of cancer have pain severe enough to be treated with opioid analgesics (Portenoy 1990). The right combination of nonpharmacologic techniques and therapeutic agents can control pain for 85 to 95 percent of patients (Abrahm 1999; Foley 1999).

Principles of Pain Management

Certain general principles are important in the evaluation of a patient's complaint of pain. Failure to follow these principles is a major cause for poor pain control.

- Believe the patient's complaint of pain. On occasion, it is necessary to ask family members or other caregivers to corroborate the patient's report of pain. When there is doubt, it is best to trust the patient.

  Ask the patient to assess the severity of the pain using pain-intensity scales. These scales often use word descriptions (0 = "no pain" to 4 = "excruciating pain") or visual analogs (a horizontal line starting with "no pain" and ending with "worst pain") whereby the patient indicates his or her perception of the pain (fig. 6.1).

  In addition to the visual analog scales, several other, more sophisticated instruments are available to measure pain. The McGill Pain Questionnaire (MPQ) is one of the most widely used tools for assessing pain. It instructs patients to make relevant selections from a list of 78 adjectives used to describe pain. An analysis of a patient's response helps the physician to determine the extent to which the

Visual Analog Scale

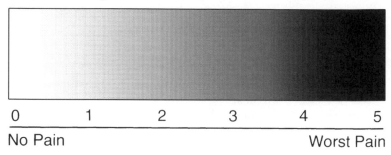

| 0 | 1 | 2 | 3 | 4 | 5 |

No Pain   Worst Pain

Figure 6.1. A visual analog scale for assessing pain

pain is mainly sensory, affective, or evaluative. The MPQ also provides a schematic body figure, which the patient shades to indicate where the pain is located. Other more practical and clinically useful tools for assessing pain include the (Wisconsin) Brief Pain Inventory (BPI) and the Memorial Pain Assessment Card (MPAC). The BPI is self-administered and requires little time to complete. Features of the BPI include graphic representation of the location of the pain, groups of qualitative descriptors, visual analog scales to measure the severity of the pain, and a perceived level of interference with normal function. The MPAC is a simple, efficient, and valid pain-assessment instrument that provides rapid clinical evaluation. Scales for quantifying the intensity of the pain, relief from pain, and mood and a set of descriptive adjectives are part of the MPAC. The MPAC is intended to help physicians distinguish the intensity of the pain, relief, and psychological distress (Rowlingson, Hamill, and Patt 1993). Physicians often tend to underestimate the patient's perception of pain (Peteet et al. 1986; Cleeland et al. 1994).

- Elicit a careful history of the pain. Inquire into when the pain occurs; its intensity, duration, character, and anatomical site(s); and its precipitating and alleviating factors. The intensity of pain is quantified using one of the previously described pain intensity scales by the physicians and caregivers. In this fashion, serial scores can determine objective changes in the patient's perception of pain as various therapeutic maneuvers are tried.
- Assess for psychological and social factors confounding the patient's expression of pain. For example, certain cultures emphasize the importance of stoicism, and patients steeped in those cultures rarely complain of pain, since this is viewed as a weakness. Other major impediments to good pain control are social factors, a common one be-

ing the family-patient dynamics regarding the ownership of pain. Failure to recognize this problem often results in convoluted and fragmented pain management. Avoidance of this is best accomplished by remembering the first principle: believe the patient's complaint of pain.

• Perform a careful medical and neurologic examination in addition to reviewing the results of various diagnostic procedures. The wizardry of modern medical technology notwithstanding, bedside examination of the patient is critical in diagnosing the etiology of pain. Understanding the limits of the diagnostic procedures is also important. To illustrate, in patients with multiple myeloma, the bone scan is often normal, whereas the bone survey frequently demonstrates the presence of osteolytic bone lesions.

• Evaluate the extent of the disease. Patients with advanced disease, regardless of the etiology, are more apt to have pain-related problems than are those with earlier disease.

• Manage the pain symptoms during the assessment to facilitate the diagnostic work-up. Allowing patients to suffer from pain during evaluation procedures is no longer acceptable. Patients may experience pain during the evaluation and also often be subjected to additional discomfort as part of the work-up (procedure pain). This procedure pain, in turn, acts as another complicating variable. In addition, a placebo should not be used to expedite the evaluation of pain.

• Diagnose the etiology of the pain, then outline and initiate a therapeutic approach. Pain is a symptom, not a diagnosis. Thus, it is critical to delineate the underlying cause of the pain. Once this step is accomplished, a therapeutic approach can be outlined and started. To prevent potential conflict, it is extremely important that the patient and family agree with this approach.

• Assess pain continuously with treatment. As previously noted, the use of a pain- assessment instrument, by both the patient and the caregiver, is very helpful in measuring the effects of the therapeutic interventions.

Finally, pain assessment is an ongoing, continuous process. The etiologies of pain often change in a patient during the course of the disease, frequently necessitating a change in treatment.

The Ladder Approach

The World Health Organization (WHO) Cancer Pain Relief program advocated the use of an analgesic ladder as a guide to the management

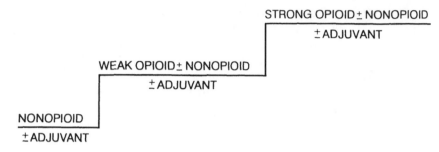

Figure 6.2. The World Health Organization analgesic ladder

of cancer pain (Jacox et al. 1994). This approach starts with nonopioid drugs, such as acetaminophen and the nonsteroidal anti-inflammatory drugs, for mild to moderate pain. If the pain persists, the next step is to use a weak opioid, like codeine or oxycodone. If no pain relief is obtained, use a strong opioid, morphine. (Patients with severe pain go straight to the top of the ladder for treatment with a strong opioid.) At each step of the ladder, adjuvant analgesics may be used (fig. 6.2).

The WHO ladder provides a rational and logical approach to pain management, and it is applicable not only to cancer but also to all areas where pain control is needed.

THE USE OF NONOPIOID ANALGESICS

Nonopioid analgesics are the first-line agents for the management of mild to moderate pain. This group includes acetaminophen and the nonsteroidal anti-inflammatory drugs (NSAIDs), such as aspirin, ibuprofen, fenoprofen, and naproxen (table 6.1). These drugs are commonly used orally, and tolerance and physical dependence do not occur with repeated administration. However, the analgesic effectiveness of the nonopioid drugs is limited by a ceiling effect, that is, escalation of the dosage beyond a certain level does not produce additional analgesia. This ceiling is usually identified by slow escalation of the dosage and may vary from patient to patient. Guidelines, which are largely empiric, for the use of NSAIDs follow.

- Select the drug. NSAIDs are useful for mild to moderate pain and often provide additive analgesia when combined with opioids in the treatment of severe pain. They may be especially useful for patients with bone pain or pain associated with inflammatory lesions. Gastrointestinal irritation and ulceration as well as bleeding due to

TABLE 6.1   The Nonopioid Analgesics

Drug	Half-life (h)	Starting Oral Dose (mg/24h)	Maximum Oral Dose (mg/24h)	Duration of Effect (h)
p-Aminophenol derivatives				
Acetaminophena	2–4	1,400	6000[e]	4–6
Salicylates				
Aspirin	3–5	1,400	6,000[e]	4–6
Diflunisal	8–12	1,000 as loading dose, then 500 every 12h	1500	8–12
Choline magnesium trisalicylate[a]	9–17	1,500 as loading dose, then 1,000 every 12h	4,000	8–12
Salsalate[a]	8–12	1,500 as loading dose, then 1,000 every 12h	4,000	8–12
Propionic acids				
Ibuprofen	1.8–2.5	1,200	4,200[e]	4–6
Naproxen	12–15	500	1,000	≤7
Naproxen sodium	12–15	550	1,100	≤7
Fenoprofen	2–3	800	3,200	4–6
Ketoprofen	2–4	150	300	6–8
Oxaprozin	40	600	1,800	24
Indoles				
Indomethacin	4.5–6	75	200	4–6
Tolmetin	1–1.5	600	2,000	6–8
Sulindac	8–16	300	400	8–12
Diclofenac	2	75	200	6
Etodolac	7	600	1,200	8
Bromfenac	1–2	75	150	6–8
Fenamates				
Mefenamic acid[b]	2–4	500 as loading dose, then 250 every 6h	1,000	6
Meclofenamate	0.5–2	150	400	6–8
Oxicams				
Piroxicam[c]	0–86	20	40[e]	48–72
Pyrazoles				
Phenylbutazone[d]	50–100	300	400	6–8
Naphthyl-alkanones				
Nabumetone	24	1,000	1,000–2,000	24

Sources: Enck (1992); Portenoy (1998).

[a]Fewer gastrointestinal and hematologic side effects.

[b]Not recommended for use more than one week; therefore, not appropriate for chronic pain management.

[c]Dosage of 40 mg per day for three weeks is associated with a high incidence of peptic ulcer, especially in older patients.

[d]Associated with the risk of severe bone marrow suppression and not preferred for chronic pain treatment.

[e]Doses that exceed the recommended daily dose may be necessary in some cases.

platelet dysfunction are the best-known toxicities associated with
NSAIDs. Often these side effects limit the clinical utility of NSAIDs
for the management of chronic pain.

- Investigate the dose-response relationship. Doses of NSAIDs should
  be initially low and then slowly be increased, at weekly intervals, to
  try to identify the ceiling dose. For older patients, the starting dose
  should be one-half to two-thirds the recommended dose. The lack of
  further analgesia after a dose increment suggests that the ceiling has
  been reached and the dose can be lowered to the previous level. Because of the dose-related toxicity of the NSAIDs, a maximal dose of
  1.5 to 2 times the standard recommended dose is suggested in ex-
  ploring the dose-response curve.
- Determine the length of the trial. In chronic cancer pain, the trial
  duration is usually a week or two; however, for other chronic diseases
  it sometimes takes weeks of treatment to determine the efficacy.
- Change to another NSAID if necessary. Because of individual variation, if one NSAID does not produce adequate analgesia, try another.
  Before changing to a different NSAID, it is critical that the clinician
  ensure that the patient has been compliant in taking the drug.

THE USE OF OPIOID ANALGESICS

After the ceiling effect is reached, drug-related toxicity occurs, or disease progression is evident by changing pain control, the opioid analgesics are the next step. These drugs, used for moderate to severe pain,
are characterized by their complex interaction with multiple opioid receptors in the nervous system. The opioid-agonist drugs, such as morphine, bind to specific opioid receptors, producing analgesia. The opioid-
antagonist drugs block the effect of morphine at its receptor. Between
these two groups are the mixed agonist-antagonist drugs, which, depending on the circumstances, demonstrate either agonist or antagonist
properties (tables 6.2 and 6.3).

TABLE 6.2   The Pharmacologic Effects of the Opioids at Receptor Sites

Mu Receptor	Kappa Receptor	Sigma Receptor
Supraspinal analgesia	Spinal analgesia	Dysphoria
Respiratory depression	Miosis	Psychomotor stimulation
Euphoria	Marked sedation	Hallucinations
Physical dependence		
Moderate sedation		

Sources: Lipman (1989); Lindley, Dalton, and Fields (1990).

Table 6.3   The Relative Activities of the Opioids at Receptor Sites

Drug	Mu Receptor	Kappa Receptor	Sigma Receptor
Morphinelike agonists	High activity	Moderate activity	Minimal to no activity
Mixed agonists-antagonists	No activity	High to moderate activity	High to low activity
Partial agonists	Moderate activity	Minimal activity	Minimal to no activity
Antagonist	High activity	High activity	Minimal activity

Sources: Lipman (1989); Lindley, Dalton, and Fields (1990).

The morphinelike agonists are the most widely used drugs to manage cancer pain. Of the opioids, oral morphine is the drug of choice. Although meperidine is a morphinelike agonist, it is not appropriate for the chronic treatment of cancer pain. Long-term administration of meperidine results in the accumulation of its metabolite, normeperidine, which causes central nervous system excitation (Lipman 1989). Also, care must be taken when using methadone. Because of its long half-life (15 to 30 hours), chronic methadone dosing can lead to drug accumulation with the clinical results of oversedation and, rarely, coma. Caution is recommended when switching from any opioid to methadone (Ripamonti et al. 1998).

The mixed agonist-antagonist drugs produce analgesia in the nontolerant patient but will precipitate withdrawal in patients tolerant to morphinelike drugs. Therefore, when these drugs are used, they should be tried before repeated administration of an opioid agonist. Because the incidence and severity of psychotomimetic side effects increase with escalation of the dosage and because only pentazocine is available in an oral preparation, these drugs play a very limited role in the management of chronic pain.

The partial agonist buprenorphine also may precipitate withdrawal in patients tolerant to morphinelike agonist and, like the mixed agonist-antagonist, should be used before the opioidlike agonist. Unlike the mixed agonist-antagonists, buprenorphine does not cause the psychotomimetic side effects. However, buprenorphine is available only in a parenteral form.

Guidelines for the use of opioid analgesics, which emphasize the individualization of therapy, follow.

• Avoid dosing "as needed" (prn). Dosing "as needed" (prn) causes a "peak and trough" effect on the blood levels of the drug, which results in uneven analgesia (fig. 6.3). Round-the-clock dosing, on the other hand, provides a constant, unfluctuating blood level of the

PRN (as needed)

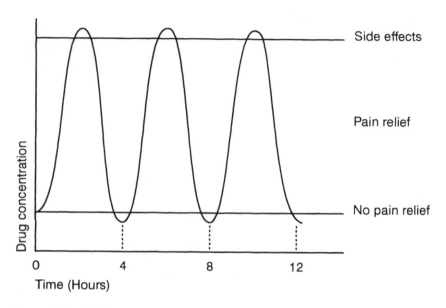

Figure 6.3. Dosing "as needed" (prn)

analgesic (Figure 6.4). Start with the lowest possible dose and titrate upward.

- Know the pharmacology of the drug used. Select and be comfortable with the use of one or two opioids. See table 6.4 for details relating to the pharmacology of the opioids.
- Choose the route of administration that maximizes the analgesic effect. The oral route is preferred for overall convenience and comfort, but occasionally other routes, such as parenteral, mucosal, intrathecal, or transdermal, are necessary.
- Use drug combinations that enhance analgesia. Combinations providing additive analgesia may reduce side effects and limit the dose escalation of the opioid component in the combination. For example, codeine combined with acetaminophen provides effective additive analgesia.
- Avoid drug combinations that increase sedation without enhancing analgesia (e.g., the empiric use of phenothiazines with morphine).
- Anticipate, recognize, and treat side effects appropriately. Side effects of opioids are either related to the central nervous system (sedation, nausea and vomiting, agitation, respiratory depression)

Round the Clock

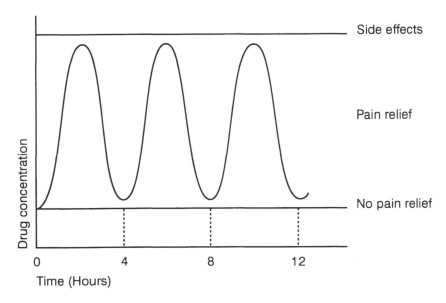

Figure 6.4. Round-the-clock dosing

or not (dry mouth, constipation, sweating, itching, urinary retention).

• Watch for the development of tolerance, and manage appropriately. Tolerance, or the need for escalating doses of opioids to maintain adequate analgesia, seems to occur in all patients receiving opioids chronically. Treat the patient who develops tolerance by switching to an alternative opioid analgesic. Due to incomplete cross-tolerance, patients who become tolerant to one opioid can be switched to another opioid to provide better analgesia. One-half of the calculated equianalgesic dose of the new drug is recommended in titrating the initial dose.

• Prevent acute withdrawal by tapering the drugs slowly and using naloxone cautiously with patients on chronic opioids.

• Respect and expect individual differences in pain and response to therapy. Older patients are more sensitive to the opioid analgesics and respond to morphine as though they had received three or four times the normal dose given to younger patients (Kaiko et al. 1982). They may receive inadequate pain control in part because of underestimation or under-reporting of pain (Bernabei et al. 1998). Also,

TABLE 6.4 The Opioid Analgesics

Drug	Equianalgesic Dose (mg)	Half-life (h)	Starting Oral Dose (mg)	Peak Effect (h)[c]	Duration (h)
Morphinelike agonists					
Morphine	10 IM[a]	2–3	30–60[b]	0.5–1.0	3–6
	60 PO[b]			1.5–2.0	4–7
Controlled-release morphine	20–60 PO	2–3	60–90	3–4	8–12
Hydromorphone	1.5 IM	2–3	4–8	0.5–1.0	3–4
	7.5 PO			1–2	3–4
Oxymorphone	1 IM	2–3	—	0.5–1	3–6
	10 PR			1.5–3	4–6
Methadone	10 IM	15–30	5–10	0.5–1.5	4–6
	20 PO			1.5–2.0	6–8
Meperidine	75 IM	2–3	75	0.5–1	3–4
	300 PO			1–2	3–6
Levorphanol	2 IM	12–16	2–4	0.5–1.0	4–6
	4 PO			1.5–2.0	4–7
Codeine	130 IM	2–3	60	1.5–2.0	3–6
	200 PO				
Oxycodone	15 IM	2–3	5	1	3–6
	30 PO				
Controlled-release oxycodone	30 PO	2–3	10–20	3–4	8–12
Hydrocodone	Available only in combination	2–4	—	0.5–1	3–4
Propoxyphene HCl	130 PO	12	65–130	1.5–2	3–6
Propoxyphene naprylate	130 PO	12	65–130	1.5–2	3–6
Fentanyl[d]	—	16–24	—	—	48–72
Mixed agonists-antagonists					
Pentazocine	60 IM	2–3	30–60	0.5–1	3–6
	180 PO			1–2	3–6
Nalbuphine	10 IM	4–6	Not available	0.5–1	3–6
Butorphanol	2 IM	2–3	Not available	0.5–1	3–4
Partial agonists					
Buprenorphine	0.4 IM	2–5	Not available	0.5–1	4–6
	0.8 SL			2–3	5–6

Sources: Enck (1992); Portenoy (1998).

[a]Morphine 10 mg IM is standard of comparison for equianalgesia.

[b]Relative potency of IM:PO morphine is 1:6 for acute pain. This ratio changes to 1:2–3 with chronic dosing.

[c]Onset of action of these drugs is generally 15 to 30 minutes.

[d]Transdermal system.

IM, intramuscular; PO, oral; PR, per rectum; SL, sublingual.

older patients are more susceptible to the side effects of both the NSAIDs and the opioids.

The Use of Adjuvant Analgesic Drugs

Adjuvant analgesic agents represent the third group of drugs used to treat chronic pain. These drugs produce analgesia by mechanisms not clearly known and not directly related to the opioid receptor system. Adjuvant analgesics include anticonvulsants, phenothiazines, antidepressants, antihistamines, steroids, and antibiotics (table 6.5). The benzodiazepines and cocaine do not provide additive analgesics to patients receiving opioids. Guidelines for the use of adjuvant analgesics follow.

- Choose a drug to match the clinical indication. The anticonvulsants, phenytoin and carbamazepine, and the tricyclic antidepressants (TCAs) are useful in managing pain of neuropathic origin, such as postherpetic neuralgia and brachial and lumbosacral plexopathy. Methotrimeprazine, a phenothiazine, produces significant analgesia independent of the opioid receptors and, therefore, does not cause significant constipation and respiratory depression. Because of these properties, methotrimeprazine is helpful for patients tolerant to opioids. Also, intermittent methotrimeprazine is useful for pain control for patients with intestinal obstruction, in whom opioids only add to the problem of obstruction. Steroids, predominantly dexamethasone, are indicated for the relief of pain due to nervous system involvement by tumor. Examples of this include brain metastases, spinal cord compression, and peripheral nerve or plexus infiltration with tumor. Finally, antibiotics may aid pain relief in certain clinical situations, most notably head and neck tumors with ulcerating tumors and pain (Bruera and MacDonald 1986).
- Understand the drug and dosage. Analgesia, for example, occurs with the TCAs at a lower dose than needed for the mood-elevating effect.
- Be aware of new or heightened side effects. Dry mouth and confusion can occur with use of the TCAs. These complications are also commonly encountered in patients receiving opioids.
- Use adjuvant analgesic drugs for a finite period of time. Antibiotics should be stopped after the signs of acute infection have resolved, generally in one to two weeks. Likewise, TCAs should be discontinued after a trial of four to six weeks if no pain-relieving effect is evident.

TABLE 6.5 The Adjuvant Analgesic Drugs

Drug	Starting Oral Dose (mg/24hr)	Indications for Use
Anticonvulsants		
Phenytoin[a]	100 initially, then slowly titrated to 300	Neuropathic pain, such as postherapetic neuralgia
Carbamazepine[a]	100 initially, then increased to 800 over a period of 7–10 days	Neuropathic pain
Gabapentin	300[b]	Neuropathic pain, especially, diabetic neuropathy and postherpetic neuralgia
Phenothiazines		
Methotrimeprazine	Not available orally 5–15 IM[c]	Opioid-tolerant patients, or to avoid opioid-induced constipation or respiratory depression
Antidepressants		
Amitriptyline	10 for older patients (25 for	Neuropathic pain others), then slowly increased to 50–75 at bedtime
Paroxetine	20	Diabetic neuropathy
Antihistamines		
Hydroxyzine[d]	25–100	Additive analgesia in combination with opioid
Steroids		
Dexamethasone	16	Nervous system involvement with or compression by tumor
Prednisone	40	
Antibiotics[e]	[e]	Acute infection associated with malignant ulceration

Sources: Enck (1992); Jacox et al. (1994); Portenoy (1998).
[a]The minimal effective dose for analgesia is not known.
[b]Lower doses may be necessary in the elderly or medically frail.
[c]15 mg IM of methotrimeprazine equivalent to 10 mg IM morphine.
[d]Anecdotal observation of usefulness based on clinical practice.
[e]Depending on organism identified and/or empiric trial.

Managing the Complications of Pain Treatment

All three groups of drug (nonopioid, opioid, and adjuvant analgesic) used to treat chronic pain have the potential to produce clinically significant side effects.

- Be proactive rather than reactive. Constipation is a frequent problem with the use of opioid analgesics. Therefore, when a patient starts taking an opioid, he or she should also start a bowel regimen such as a daily stool softener and laxative to lessen this side effect.
- Recognize and treat side effects appropriately. The major effect of the opioids on the central nervous system is sedation or drowsiness. This may be managed by reducing the drug dosage and prescribing the drug more frequently or by switching to an analgesic with a shorter half-life. Generally, amphetamines are not useful for enhancing the comfort of terminally ill patients. In some instances, however, they are able to decrease sedation and increase activity by offsetting the opioid side effects (Bruera et al. 1987d). Nausea and vomiting are managed by either changing the patient to an alternative opioid or using an antiemetic, such as a phenothiazine or an antihistamine. In some instances, tolerance to nausea develops and the antiemetics can be tapered. As previously mentioned, these drugs, especially the phenothiazines, can potentiate the sedating effect of the opioids.

   Respiratory depression is potentially the most serious side effect of opioid therapy. It usually occurs with the acute administration of morphine to an opioid-naive patient. Rarely, patients being treated chronically with opioids develop respiratory depression. Slowly give diluted naloxone (an opioid antagonist) intravenously, and titrate carefully to prevent the precipitation of acute withdrawal symptoms.
- Prevent acute opioid withdrawal. Physical dependence is a pharmacologic effect of opioids. Withdrawal symptoms occur when the drug is stopped and are prevented by slowly tapering the drug over the course of one to two weeks. As noted above, the clinician should prescribe naloxone carefully for patients treated with opioids on a chronic basis.
- Avoid polypharmacy. For example, the use of steroids with the NSAIDs has the serious potential to increase not only gastrointestinal irritation but also the risk for bleeding. Confusion and other central nervous system toxicities are seen not only with the opioids but also with the NSAIDs and some adjuvant analgesics. Exercise care to avoid additive side effects due to indiscriminate combination of these drugs.

• Consider alternative pain control therapies if side effects are un-manageable or intolerable. If the pain is not relieved pharmacolog-ically, consider other therapeutic interventions.

Summary

Guidelines on evaluating a patient's complaint of pain; on the use of nonopioid, opioid, and adjuvant analgesic drugs; and on managing the complications of pain treatment are readily available to physicians. No new drugs or treatment methods are needed, only enlightenment and further education by physicians, to provide good-quality care to dying pa-tients. Past concerns about addicting patients to opioid analgesics are sci-entifically unfounded. Using appropriate doses of opioid analgesics, such as morphine, for the severe pain of cancer and other chronic diseases is simply good care.

Chapter 7

Opioids

Oral Morphine

Of all the natural and synthetic opioids, oral morphine is the standard for comparison and is the drug of choice for chronic severe pain (McQuay 1999). Orally administered morphine is subject to the first-pass effect of liver metabolism (glucuronidation), which causes a large reduction in its potency. In a single-dose study, Sawe et al. (1981) investigated the kinetics of both oral and intravenous morphine in seven cancer patients. They found a 15 to 64 percent variation in oral bioavailability, with a mean of 38 percent. In addition, they showed a marked interindividual variation in the terminal half-life, from 58 to 467 minutes. This unique wide individual variation in the metabolism of morphine accounts for the broad range of therapeutic doses, which may vary from only 30 mg a day to several grams a day to achieve good relief of pain (Hoskin and Hanks 1990).

The intramuscular (IM) administration of morphine at a dose of 10 mg is considered the standard for comparison to other dosages and other opioid analgesics. Morphine given in this manner and dose produces an onset of action at 20 to 60 minutes, with a peak effect at 30 to 60 minutes and a three-to six-hour duration. For a similar but slightly larger effect, the oral dose is 60 mg for acute pain and 20 to 30 mg for chronic administration (Berry 1988). This difference in oral:parenteral potency from 6:1 in acute dosing versus 2–3:1 for chronic dosing is thought to be due to the accumulation of the pharmacologically active metabolite morphine-6-glucuronide (M6G) (Weissman, Dahl, and Joranson 1990).

Clinically, the use of oral morphine remains empiric. The usual starting dose for an opioid-naive patient is 20 to 30 mg every four hours. The most important factor determining the dose required is the severity of the pain. As reported by Hoskin and Hanks (1990), a retrospective analysis of clinical data from cancer patients indicates that age is also a predictor of dose, with patients under 60 years old having a median maximum (four hourly) dose requirement of 55 mg, compared with only 25 to 30 mg for those over 60 years old. Pharmacokinetic differences for morphine in different age groups have been found, with a reduced clearance and smaller volume of distribution in older patients.

Morphine has an active metabolite, M6G, which is a major metabolite and is more potent than morphine. An unexpected degree and duration of effect of M6G can occur in patients with severely impaired renal function who are given morphine. Drug doses should be reduced substantially if the creatinine clearance is less than 30 mL/min per 1.73 m2. With less severe renal function, careful titration of the dosage is necessary, especially for older patients. The glucuronidation of morphine is not significantly affected in cirrhosis, but the kinetics and dynamics of morphine metabolism are altered in pre-hepatic coma states (McQuay 1999). Factors affecting the enterohepatic circulation of morphine, such as cholestasis, bowel resection, and the use of antibiotics, have not shown a meaningful effect on the overall dose requirements.

The issue of opioid rotation, that is, changing from morphine to a different opioid due to inadequate analgesia, is unclear. For those patients for whom further escalation of the dosage is not possible because of toxicity, rotating to another opioid offers the advantage of lowering the dosage while achieving better pain contol because of incomplete cross-tolerance (Payne 1999). On the other hand, McQuay (1999) favored changing the route of opioid administration (i.e., route rotation), rather than changing the drug. He noted that until there are more hard data that a genuine advantage exists in changing a drug, such as a differential rate of adverse effects or evidence from a randomized comparison of the two strategies, the issue remains unresolved.

After the pain has been controlled and a 24-hour dose of morphine has been determined, treatment can be continued with an immediate-release preparation (4-hour dosing) alone. Alternatively, a long-acting/controlled-release preparation (12-hour dosing) can be started using an immediate-release morphine for breakthrough pain.

CONTROLLED-RELEASE ORAL MORPHINE

Although controlled-release oral morphine preparations have been available in the United States for some time, the use of these products has been a source of confusion and misunderstanding by caregivers, especially physicians. This problem was highlighted in a study by White et al. (1991), who sought to assess prescribing practices for patients with cancer pain among populations of physicians in the United Kingdom. A postal questionnaire was sent to every member of the medical staff in four different types of medical practice to try to provide a broad view of physicians' attitudes. These practices included a specialist oncology hospital, an undergraduate teaching hospital, a general hospital, and general practitioners in both inner city and suburban areas.

Overall, the response rate to the questionnaire was 42 percent (265/625). The drug of first choice for analgesia for patients with severe cancer pain was morphine: 66 percent of physicians chose it. Further analysis of this group showed that 20 percent prescribed a morphine elixir and 46 percent preferred a controlled-release morphine (MST Continus) preparation. The use of this controlled-release product was particularly popular among general practitioners and younger physicians. MST was also chosen by 56 percent of physicians with no oncology experience but by only 30 percent of those with more than three years experience in oncology.

The vast majority of respondents (93%) indicated that they would administer their drug of first choice regularly, and 84 percent chose the oral route as their first choice of administration. Of the physicians who preferred MST, 63 percent would administer the drug at 12-hour intervals, while 37 percent indicated that they would use the drug at less than 12-hour intervals. Of the entire group of responding physicians, only 17 percent choosing morphine defined an upper dose limit; of these, 12 percent used MST as the preferred formulation.

In this study, most physicians chose morphine as their first-choice analgesic, 84 percent chose the oral route, and 87 percent indicated that they would administer the analgesic on a regular basis. Morphine elixir was the formulation of choice in the specialist oncology hospital, but controlled-release morphine tablets (MST) were the preferred form in both other hospitals and general practice. MST was clearly preferred by those with less than five years of experience. MST was prescribed in regimens varying from once a day to every 2 hours. As noted by the authors, this indicates considerable confusion about controlled-release morphine. Although the awareness of the preparation is very high, the drug appears to be subject to widespread misuse. MST is designed for 12-hourly administration and infrequently has to be given more often.

A well-known principle in the use of morphine for pain due to advanced cancer is that there is no arbitrary upper limit of the dose, since morphine has no ceiling effect. A minority of the respondents in this study did indicate an upper dose limit and, in many cases, at a fairly modest level. It is notable that a majority of these physicians used MST as their preferred formulation. There is little doubt that, if this survey were done in the United States, similar misperceptions regarding controlled-release morphine preparations would be identified in U.S. physicians.

Because oral morphine has a short half-life, peak effect, and duration, it must be administered every 4 hours to achieve optimal effect. Unfortunately, a 4-hour regimen is inconvenient for patients because it requires dosing during the night. In addition, compliance is known to decrease as the required frequency of dosing increases, and noncompliance adds to the risk of suboptimal pain control.

In a study of pharmacokinetics and clinical efficacy, Thirlwell et al. (1989) compared an oral morphine solution given every 4 hours to a controlled-release morphine tablet (MS Contin) administered every 12 hours in 23 adult patients with chronic pain due to cancer. The steady-state plasma concentration versus time profile obtained with cancer patients taking MS Contin every 12 hours demonstrated that the prolonged release of morphine from tablets reduced both the rate of absorption and the rate of decline of plasma morphine concentrations. As suggested by the authors, these pharmacokinetics indicate that a 12-hour regimen of MS Contin should be optimal for most patients. Although plasma concentrations of morphine were declining at the end of the 12-hour period, at no time did they fall significantly below the corresponding concentrations achieved with the morphine solution. This finding parallels the clinical observation that there is no loss of analgesic efficacy over the last few hours of the MS Contin dose interval.

Furthermore, Thirlwell et al. (1989) confirmed what others (Hanks 1989) had reported, namely, that 12-hour dosing with controlled-release morphine produces pain control equivalent to that achieved with a 4-hour regimen. They also suggested a daily milligram equivalency when transferring patients from oral morphine preparations to controlled-release formulations such as MS Contin.

Clearly, controlled-release morphine is for maintenance treatment once the patient's morphine requirement has been determined, and it is inappropriate for administration "as required." The pattern of adverse effects with these formulations seems to be similar to that of conventional oral morphine preparations. However, there may be some advantage in the quality of sleep with controlled-release morphine, possibly related to fewer fluctuations in plasma and central nervous system concentrations of morphine and its metabolites (Hanks 1989).

In a randomized, double-blind, cross-over trial, Bruera et al. (1998) compared the safety and efficacy of oral controlled-release oxycodone with that of controlled-release morphine in 32 patients with cancer pain. Twenty-three of the 32 patients enrolled completed the study and were evaluable. The mean 24-hour dose was 93 mg for controlled-release oxycodone (OxyContin) versus 145 mg for controlled-release morphine (MS Contin). There were no significant differences demonstrated between the two treatments in pain intensity, sedation, nausea, frequency and mean severity of adverse events, clinical effectiveness scores, or patient and investigator preference scores. The authors found that initial dose ratios of 2:1 or higher should be used when converting from controlled-release morphine to controlled-release oxycodone to allow for incomplete cross-tolerance. They concluded that controlled-release oxycodone is as safe and effective as controlled-release morphine in the treatment of cancer pain.

Finally, Mansour, Abdel-Rahman, and Wold (1999) retrospectively reviewed the use of controlled-release morphine and oxycodone in 111 patients treated in a hospice in 1997. The mean daily doses prescribed for controlled-release morphine (MS Contin) and controlled-release oxycodone (OxyContin) were 692.4 mg (range of 30 to 7,800 mg) and 93.6 mg (range of 20 to 1,020 mg), respectively. The authors hoped that this information on very high average doses of controlled-release opioids would be helpful to others in achieving pain relief for terminally ill cancer patients.

Parenteral Opioids

Treatment with parenteral opioids is especially useful for patients who cannot tolerate the oral route. Studies of pain management show that the majority of patients require at least two routes of administration (oral and parenteral) during the course of their painful disease and that one-third require at least three alternative routes (Coyle et al. 1990).

CONTINUOUS INTRAVENOUS INFUSIONS

The continuous intravenous (IV) infusion of opioid analgesics has been used in the management of both postoperative pain and chronic cancer pain. One study of 210 dying patients treated during a two-year period revealed that 13 percent received a continuous IV infusion of morphine before death (Kellar 1984). In 1986, Portenoy et al. published the results of a three-year retrospective review of their experience with continuous IV infusions with hospitalized cancer patients of the Pain Service at Memorial Sloan-Kettering Cancer Center. Forty-six infusions in 36 patients were identified for study. These 46 infusions accounted for approximately 3 percent of Pain Service consultations during the three-year period.

The median age of the 36 patients was 42 years, with a range of 1.5 to 67 years. All patients had received opioids before starting infusions, with wide variation in the quantity of opioids consumed during the 24 hours preceding the infusions. Morphine was the most frequently infused drug (36 patients), followed by methadone (4), hydromorphone (4), oxymorphone (1), and levorphanol (1). In morphine equivalents, the mean starting dose was 17 mg/hour, the mean maximum infusion rate was 69 mg/ hour, and the mean rate of infusion termination was 52 mg/hour. The duration of the infusions varied from 1 to 45 days.

Pain relief was defined as acceptable if the patient remained awake and coherent and analgesia was reported to be adequate in either nurse's or physician's notes during consecutive days after the infusion was started. Based on these criteria, pain was relieved in 61 percent of the patients, leaving 37 percent with inadequate pain control. Pain relief was indeterminate in one patient.

The authors were uncertain as to why more than one-third of the patients were unable to obtain adequate pain control with continuous IV infusion, but they offered several explanations. They noted that this phenomenon was observed most commonly in patients whose pain occurred episodically, usually with movement (incident pain), in those whose pain was due to nervous system injury that interrupted the normal transmission of sensory impulses (deafferentation pain), and in those whose pain was a component of a more global nature not amenable to treatment with opioids. Side effects were common and included sedation, confusion, nausea, and vomiting. Respiratory depression occurred in only one patient, who was also concurrently receiving intrathecal morphine. Portenoy et al. (1986) thought that the continuous IV infusion of opioids, predominantly morphine, was safe, but they recommended a trial of repetitive IV bolus dosing before initiating continuous infusion in most patients.

Based on this study, as well as others, I suggest the following indications for the use of the continuous IV infusion of opioids:

- intolerance of IM and oral routes;
- the need for frequent injections, more often than every two hours, for pain control;
- the presence of prominent bolus effects, such as sedation or the rapid return of pain after injections, on repetitive dosing; and
- the need for rapid titration (table 7.1).

TABLE 7.1   The Indications for the Continuous Intravenous Infusion of Opioids

---

Intolerance of intramuscular and oral routes
Frequent injections required
Presence of prominent bolus effects, such as sedation or the rapid
   return of pain following injections
Need for rapid titration of analgesia

Sources: Portenoy et al. (1986); Payne (1987a).

Rarely, patients require very high doses of continuous IV morphine for pain control. In a five-year retrospective review, Gregory et al. (1991) identified six patients at the Johns Hopkins Oncology Center who were treated with more than 4 grams of IV morphine per day. Three patients received this dosage for less than 24 hours without seizures. Two of the three remaining patients developed grand mal seizures on the second and third days after morphine infusions of 4.8 and 6.7 grams/day, respectively. On further study, the investigators found that IV solutions of morphine typically contained bisulfite preservatives. The usual exposure to these bisulfite preservatives was less than 100 mg/day, and higher doses, especially when given continuously, had previously been associated with seizures. Based on this, the authors postulated that prolonged IV infusion of high-dose morphine places patients at risk for seizures from the accumulation of toxic doses of bisulfite preservatives. Furthermore, they suggested that patients requiring high doses of IV opioids receive agents that are free of bisulfite preservatives.

Unfortunately, continuous IV infusions are cumbersome and expensive, are not readily transportable to the home setting, and often require a permanent central venous port (Cherny and Foley 1996). Therefore, the use of continuous subcutaneous infusions is a viable alternative.

Continuous Subcutaneous Infusions

In 1986, Coyle et al., from the Pain Service at Memorial Sloan-Kettering Cancer Center, reported their experience with 15 advanced cancer patients who were managed with the continuous subcutaneous (SC) infusion of opioids. The mean age of these patients was 54 years, with a range of 23 to 71 years. Nine of the 15 patients had either obstruction or a malabsorption syndrome, and all had prior treatment with parenteral opioids. Morphine was the most common opioid employed in 9 patients (range of 3.5 to 9.7 mg/hour), followed by hydromorphone in 3 (range of 1.0 to 7.5 mg/hour), levorphanol in 2 (range of 1.0 to 4.0 mg/hour), and methadone in 1 (range of 10.0 to 24 mg/hour). SC infusion used a portable, battery-operated infusion pump attached to a 27-gauge butterfly needle placed subcutaneously. Any SC site could be used on a rotating basis, but the subclavicular area and anterior chest wall were frequently used to permit free movement of the patient's arms and legs. The complete tubing, infusion site, and needle were routinely changed every week. Patients remained on the continuous SC infusion from 3 to 76 days. Thirteen of the 15 patients (87%) rated their pain control as good. The only complication was local irritation at the infusion site in 5 patients. The average patient underwent a change of site every three days, although one patient required this every six hours (Maouskop et al. 1985; Coyle et al. 1986).

TABLE 7.2 The Indications for the Continuous Subcutaneous Infusion of Opioids

---

Avoids the need for intravenous access
No delay in opioid administration
Continuous level of pain control without peak and trough drug levels
Readily accepted and managed by patients and their families

Sources: Coyle et al. (1986); Payne (1987a).

According to this group, the major indication for continuous SC infusion of opioids is the requirement for prolonged administration of parenteral opioids. SC infusions offer the following significant advantages over the use of intermittent SC, IM, or IV routes:

- they avoid repetitive IM/SC injections;
- they avoid the need for IV access;
- they free the patient from delay in administration of opioid analgesic;
- they provide a continuous level of pain control with no peak-level side effects or trough- level pain breakthrough;
- they are readily accepted and managed by patients and their families; and
- they allow earlier discharge home without compromising pain control (table 7.2).

However, continuous SC infusions may be impractical in patients

- who have generalized edema;
- who develop erythema, soreness, or sterile abscesses with SC administration;
- who have bleeding disorders (Expert Working Group of the European Association for Palliative Care 1996).

In another study from the Cross Cancer Institute, in Edmonton, Alberta, (Bruera et al. 1987c), 56 patients with advanced cancer were managed with continuous SC infusions of either morphine (34 patients) or hydromorphone (22 patients). Unlike the study at Memorial Sloan-Kettering Cancer Center, pain control was achieved with IV opioids before the start of the SC infusion. Another difference was the use of a non-battery-powered pump. The mean duration of infusion was 26 ± 14 days, with 45 percent of patients being discharged to home for an average of 18 days. After 48 hours of SC infusion, 96 percent preferred the SC infusion to their previous IV treatment because of increased comfort, easier mobility, and better pain control. Systemic toxicity included severe drowsiness or confusion (14%), which improved on adjustment of the dosage of the infusion. One patient (2%) developed respiratory depression, which improved with discontinuation of the hydromorphone infusion. Local toxicity consisted of infection (3%), chemical irritation (5%), and bleeding (1%). No difference was found between morphine and hydromorphone in pain control or toxicity. In addition, a subset of patients who were poor candidates for home discharge, namely those requiring frequent dose increases to maintain adequate pain control, was identified. The authors of this study concluded that SC infusion of opioid with a portable disposable device is a safe and simple method for administering effective analgesia to inpatients as well as outpatients.

Few studies directly compared the SC and IV routes of continuous infusion of opioid until the report by Moulin et al. in 1991. In a randomized, double-blind, cross-over trial, these investigators studied 53 patients with advanced cancer who had been started on continuous SC infusions of opioids because of substantial side effects from oral or rectal analgesics. Twenty patients (10 male and 10 female, with a mean age of 62 years) participated in the study, with 23 refusing and 10 excluded because of metabolic encephalopathy or brain metastases. Using SC infusions before the trial, the investigators established the maximal analgesic dose of hydormorphone with minimal side effects. For each 48-hour trial period, new infusion sites were started on the abdomen or anterior chest wall. The study was double-blind by the use of two programmable infusion pumps. During active SC infusion, the IV pump delivered saline or hydromorphone. Morphine injections were given every three hours for breakthrough pain.

Serial measurements of pain intensity, pain relief, mood, and sedation using visual analog scales showed no statistically or clinically significant differences between the two routes of infusion. The mean hydromorphone infusion rate was 6.1 mg/hour, with a range of 1 to 35 mg/hour. Side effects were minimal (four patients experienced nausea). The mean number of morphine injections for breakthrough pain during the 48-hour trial period did not differ significantly between the routes (4.8 for IV versus 5.3 for SC). The investigators used hydromorphone because of its high analgesic potency (i.e., five to six times that of morphine). This pharmacologic property minimized the volume of infusion and maximized the duration of use of each pump reservoir. These features were particularly advantageous for the home setting of continuous SC infusions. Opioid-tolerant patients requiring more than 10 mg/hour for adequate pain control needed at least a 50 mg/hour equivalent infusion of morphine, which required a specially prepared morphine solution of high concentration or a greater volume of infusion. Because of the simplicity, technical advantages, and cost-effectiveness of continuous SC infusion of opioid, the authors advocated the abandonment of the IV infusions for the management of severe cancer pain, except in rare circumstances.

PATIENT-CONTROLLED ANALGESIA

Some patients experience side effects related to intermittent high doses and breakthrough pain with oral opioids such as morphine. In well over half of these patients, the use of continuous IV or SC infusions of opioids has provided effective pain control. Therefore, the addition of a patient-controlled analgesia (PCA) system whereby patients receiving a continuous infusion of opioids could give themselves additional bolus doses was a logical extension.

PCA was initially described by Sechzer in 1968 (White 1988). At that time, he evaluated the analgesic response to small doses of IV opioid analgesics given on patient demand by a nurse-observer. Although this system provided improved pain relief with smaller total dosages, it proved impractical because of the demands it placed on nursing personnel.

In the late 1960s, researchers began testing instruments that would enable patients to self-administer small IV doses of opioids when they felt the need for them. One of the key features of these devices was the development of a lockout or delay interval. The purpose of the lockout interval was to prevent the patient from administering a second dose until after the first dose had time to exert its peak pharmacologic effect.

In 1970, investigators described an instrument that automatically administered IV analgesic drugs after the patient pressed the button on a handgrip device. In a pilot study involving 30 patients, they reported that patient and physician acceptance was good and that the safety features were reliable. The following year, Sechzer described his initial experience with a PCA system and concluded that it was a highly satisfactory method for treating postoperative pain and that good analgesia was achieved with relatively low total drug doses. In the ensuing years, multiple reports in the medical literature have shown the value of PCA in managing short-term, acute postoperative pain.

PCA is a system designed to accommodate a wide range of analgesic requirements. It can also minimize the anxiety resulting from the slow onset of pain relief associated with the most commonly used therapeutic modalities. A major psychological advantage with PCA relates to its ability to minimize the time interval between the perception of pain and the administration of an analgesic. In addition, the increased attention being paid to the PCA-treated patient might provide a psychological bene-

fit to the patient. With PCA therapy, patients experience minimal sedation during awake hours and few side effects.

In 1986, Citron et al. published the results of their study of PCA in
eight patients with cancer. This open study was to determine standard
dose ranges and lockout intervals in addition to patient acceptance of this
mode of treatment for cancer pain. The duration of each trial was no
longer than 96 hours. Respiratory rates, mental status, and pain relief
were recorded at baseline and during the study period. In some patients,
a loading dose of IV morphine was delivered by the infusion pump to provide initial pain relief. PCA doses of morphine ranged from 1 to 5 mg,
with lockout intervals from 15 to 90 minutes. The length of this lockout
interval was selected to prevent patients from having to self-administer
medication so often that it would interfere with their activity. Many of the
patients administered medication about every two hours after they
achieved their initial pain control and, in general, the patients had a
higher analgesic demand during the first four hours than during the remaining time of treatment. Respiratory rates decreased during the first
four hours of treatment, but no cases of significant respiratory depression
occurred during this period or thereafter in the study.

At the end of the study, all patients expressed satisfaction with PCA,
and five patients preferred this mode of pain control over conventional
methods of giving opioids. Concerns regarding potential opioid overdose
with PCA therapy were addressed, and the investigators noted that proper
infusion pump settings for the amount of morphine to be delivered and
the lockout interval minimized this risk. Base on their study, the authors
concluded that PCA was an effective and safe therapy for cancer pain.

Kerr et al. (1988) studied 18 patients with poorly controlled cancer
pain who were treated with both continuous infusion (IV or SC) opioid
therapy and PCA. This study differed from that of Citron et al. (1986) in
that all patients were managed in the outpatient setting. The portable infusion pump used in the study not only administered a continuous infusion of the opioid but also permitted patients to give bolus injections "as
needed."

Eighteen cancer patients completed at least one outpatient infusion of
opioids. Conventional opioid dosing was changed because of breakthrough pain in most patients (15) followed by significant side effects,
such as nausea and vomiting (6), drowsiness (4), inconvenient frequent
injection (2), and dysphagia (1). The lockout interval for the PCA was 30
to 60 minutes. Most patients received either morphine or hydromorphone. A single patient was on meperidine. The maximal doses of these
opioids were morphine, 80 mg/hour; hydromorphone, 60 mg/hour;
and meperidine, 50 mg/hour. The outpatient infusions were easily man-

ageable for long periods, with an average of 54 days and a range from 7 to 225 days. The majority of patients required some escalation of the dosage during the first 14 days. Side effects were minimal, and improved pain control was achieved by all patients.

In 1989, Swanson et al. reported the largest series of cancer patients using PCA for chronic pain. The study of these 117 patients was conducted in the setting of a private practice incorporating a community-based, multidisciplinary approach. Sixty-nine percent of the patients were treated at home, and 31 percent were managed in hospice. All patients received either an SC (87%) or an IV (13%) continuous infusion of opioid along with the capability of PCA bolus for breakthrough pain. There was a wide range in the amount of opioid required to achieve adequate analgesia: the patients on IV morphine received a larger dosage (mean of 24 mg/hour) than did those on SC infusions (mean of 6.5 mg/hour). The bolus dose of morphine was the same (4 mg) for both groups. The mean age of the patients was 61.2 years, with a preponderance of men (62%). The vast majority of patients were treated with morphine; treatment ranged from 1 to 295 days, with an average duration of therapy of 23 days. In these patients, bone pain was the most frequent complaint.

Of the 117 patients studied, 95 percent experienced pain relief after the initiation of PCA. Side effects were rare, consisting of SC needle site infection and respiratory depression. Progressive pain due to either advancing disease or the development of drug tolerance was controlled by increasing the rates of opioid infusion. The authors concluded that continuous infusion of opioids along with PCA bolus capability can be started and administered safely in the home.

PCA may be most advantageous in the management of incident pain, that is, pain that is quiescent at rest but occurs immediately with movement. In this setting, patients can premedicate themselves on anticipation of movement. Also, gaining a sense of control, which is implicit with PCA, may be of psychological benefit to patients.

Although the number of studies is small and there are no double-blind, cross-over trials, PCA appears to be effective in some subsets of patients with cancer pain. Some investigators have concerns about the overuse that is occurring because of the generalized prescription of an expensive technology such as PCA for cancer patients by simple extrapolation of data from PCA postoperative trials. More clinical studies are needed to determine the best type of opioid, as well as the ideal dose per injection and lockout interval. Issues such as circadian modulation, opioid rotation, and the relative amount of extra dose in patients receiving continuous infusion should be addressed in these studies. Less expensive and simpler devices should be developed to decrease the cost and increase the comfort of the patients, families, and nurses with this technique. Because of the expense of PCA, cost-effective studies should be conducted to ensure that this technique is properly applied (Ripamonti 1998).

Alternative Routes of Administration

Generally, the favored routes of administration of morphine are oral and parenteral. Alternatively, the sublingual, buccal, and rectal routes are useful (1) when oral morphine is impractical because of nausea, vomiting, bowel obstruction, or difficulty swallowing; and (2) when parenteral injections are difficult or painful, as in the presence of a bleeding disorder, emaciation, or inaccessible veins.

A major advantage for the alternative routes is the avoidance of the first-pass effect, resulting in a more rapid onset and longer duration of analgesia in addition to lower doses and fewer side effects (fig. 7.1). However, the use of sublingual, buccal, and rectal routes can be limited by unpalatable taste and irritation of the sublingual mucosa (table 7.3).

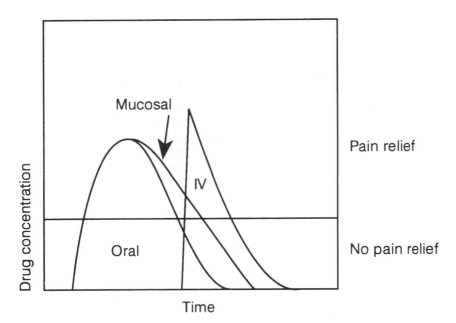

Figure 7.1. Drug concentrations versus time for oral, mucosal, and parenteral (IV) administrations of morphine

TABLE 7.3 The Advantages and
Disadvantages of Sublingual, Rectal, and Buccal
Administration of Morphine

Advantages
    Oral or parenteral routes impractical
    Avoidance of "first pass" effects
Disadvantages
    Poor bioavailability of drugs
    Unpalatable taste
    Buccal irritation

Source: Payne (1987a).

SUBLINGUAL ADMINISTRATION

Pitorak and Kraus (1987) reported their favorable experience with sublingual morphine for pain control in hospice patients. Morphine tablets were placed sublingually. This method was preferred over the liquid preparation, since there was less likelihood that the patient would swallow the medication. Occasionally, patients complained about the bitter taste of the morphine tablet. The incidence of constipation and vomiting decreased, and pain management continued on schedule despite interruptions of gastrointestinal absorption. Lower doses of morphine were required, with a usual dosage of 10 mg to 40 mg every three to four hours. This lessened dose was more cost effective: a total 24-hour dose of 60 mg cost only $0.72. Despite the very limited, albeit favorable, clinical experience with the sublingual route, the question of the bioavailability of morphine is still debated (Payne 1987a), with some (Lipman 2000) reporting that only 22 percent of morphine given via this route is absorbed.

Buprenorphine, a partial agonist with a peak and duration of effect similar to that of morphine but higher sublingual absorption (Lipman 2000), has also been reported as being efficacious for cancer pain control via the sublingual route. As reviewed by Payne (1987a), one study from England treated 141 cancer patients with sublingual buprenorphine in doses of 0.15 mg to 0.8 mg for an average of three months. This regimen was effective in the majority of patients, especially those with pain from head and neck cancers. Drowsiness was the most common side effect, but dry mouth and nausea also occurred. Constipation was not seen.

BUCCAL ADMINISTRATION

Another alternative route of administering morphine is by way of the buccal mucosa membrane. Once the morphine tablet adheres to the buccal mucosa, the uptake of the active drug is principally governed by local blood flow, as with IM injections. Buccal administration has advantages over sublingual drug delivery: the presence of the drug in the mouth is easily tolerated, and it does not stimulate salivation (which can speed the solution of the tablet so it is more easily swallowed and thus rendered less active).

In a study of postoperative analgesia, Bell et al. (1985) demonstrated the safety and effectiveness of buccal morphine. In this randomized study, buccal tablets containing 13.3 mg of morphine were placed between the upper lip and the gum above the incisor teeth in 20 patients. The tablets were usually moistened to facilitate their adherence to the mucosa, and they slowly dissolved within six hours. In another 20 patients, 13.3 mg of morphine was given in the form of IM injection. The two routes of administration produced a similar degree of postoperative analgesia, as assessed by the average reduction in pain score and the pain relief score. Peak concentrations of plasma morphine were slightly lower after buccal than after IM administration, but they declined more slowly. Consequently, the drug's bioavailability was 40 to 50 percent greater after buccal than after IM administration.

The buccal route was very acceptable to patients. Only 1 of the 20 patients complained of a bitter taste and stopped the preparation after two hours. In all patients, no untoward effects on the mucosa were noted at the site of application. Nausea, vomiting, or both, as well as dizziness or drowsiness, occurred less often in patients treated by buccal administration. Based on these findings, Bell et al. (1985) suggested that buccal morphine may be valuable in managing chronic pain due to malignant disease. Unfortunately, no large-scale study evaluating buccal morphine in this setting has been published.

Oral transmucosal fentanyl citrate (OTFC) is a new therapy to manage breakthrough pain, which occurs in about two-thirds of patients with well-controlled chronic pain (Portenoy and Lesage 1999). OTFC is a unique formulation in which fentanyl, an opioid approximately 75 times more potent than morphine, is incorporated into a sweetened lozenge attached to a stick. The fentanyl is absorbed through the buccal and sublingual mucosa as the lozenge dissolves in the mouth. OTFC has been shown to have properties of onset and peak activity similar to those of IV morphine. Of the total available dose, 25 percent is absorbed transmucosally during a 15-minute period and an additional 25 percent is absorbed through the gastrointestinal tract over the next 90 minutes. Meaningful pain relief occurs as soon as 5 minutes in patients with postoperative pain (Streisand et al. 1991; Farrar et al. 1998).

In a placebo-controlled, double-blinded, randomized trial, Farrar et al. (1998) investigated the effectiveness of OTFC for breakthrough cancer pain. The 92 patients who agreed to participate in the study had sufficient pain to require the equivalent of 60 mg/day oral morphine or at least 50 μg/hour transdermal fentanyl and had at least one episode of break-through pain per day for which they took additional opioids. The authors found that OTFC produced significantly larger changes in pain intensity and better pain relief than placebo. Dizziness, nausea, and somnolence were the most frequent side effects. In this study, OTFC appeared effective in treating cancer-related breakthrough pain.

Christie et al. (1998) studied the dose-titration of OTFC for break-through pain in cancer patients using transdermal fentanyl for chronic pain. Of the 62 patients in the study, slightly more than half were women (53%) and the median age was 59 years. The majority of patients (76%) found a safe and effective dose of OTFC for breakthrough pain. The mean successful dose of OTFC in this study was approximately 600 μg, which corresponds to a mean dose of 18 mg of oral morphine. There was no significant relationship between the around-the-clock opioid regimen and the effective dose of OTFC. In addition, OTFC produced a faster on-set and a greater degree of pain relief than patients' usual breakthrough medication. Side effects were similar to those in the study by Farrar et al. (1998), namely, somnolence, nausea, and dizziness. According to this study, most patients find that a single dose of OTFC adequately treats breakthrough pain and that the optimal dose is found by titration and is not predicted by the around-the-clock dose of opioids.

RECTAL ADMINISTRATION

The third alternative for administering morphine is rectally. During a five-year period (1980–85), Steitz (1987), from Connecticut Hospice, re-ported an increase in the use of rectal administration from 2.2 percent (1980–81) to 6.5 percent (1984–85). This increase was attributed to bet-ter availability of suppository dosage forms of morphine.

Ellison and Lewis (1984) compared 10-mg doses of morphine in oral solution and rectal suppository in a single-dose pharmacokinetic study. They found that morphine was better absorbed from a rectal suppository than from oral solution. In addition, plasma concentrations of morphine were significantly higher during the 4.5-hour time span measured after the rectal suppository than after the oral solution. The authors empha-sized that these results cannot be generalized to patients receiving mul-tiple daily doses of morphine, which is the usual clinical occurrence.

Maloney et al. (1989) described a novel use for controlled-release mor-phine (MS Contin) via the rectal route. All 39 of their terminally ill pa-tients had good pain control but were unable to take oral medication be-cause of intractable nausea, inability to swallow, or both. MS Contin

30-mg tablets were administered rectally for periods of 1 to 30 days, with a mean of 11.5 days. The dose range was 2 to 30 tablets daily, with a mean of 6.2 tablets. Sixteen patients were maintained on an every-12-hour schedule, 17 patients on an 8-hour schedule, and 6 patients on a 6-hour schedule. Pain control was maintained in all patients. In 11 patients, the dose of MS Contin was decreased. No local or systemic adverse reactions developed. In terminally ill patients, the rectal administration of tablets of MS Contin was a safe, effective, and simple method of maintaining good pain control.

In a subsequent study, Bruera et al. (1995) confirmed the efficacy and safety of rectally administered controlled-release morphine in cancer patients. Thirty patients with cancer pain were randomized in a double-blind, cross-over study to receive either controlled-release morphine suppositories every 12 hours or SC morphine every 4 hours for 4 days. No significant differences were observed between the controlled-release suppositories and SC morphine in overall pain intensity, sedation, nausea, or daily rescue analgesic consumption. The authors thought that controlled-release suppositories are a safe and effective noninvasive alternative to parenteral morphine for patients who are unable to take oral medications because of nausea, vomiting, dysphagia, bowel obstruction, or severe confusion.

Finally, in a related study, DeConno et al. (1995) randomized 34 opioid-naive patients with cancer to receive morphine hydrochloride 10 mg either orally or rectally for 2 days. A cross-over occurred at days 3 and 4. Every 10 minutes, for a total of 240 minutes, pain, nausea, and sedation were assessed. Rectal morphine was found to have a faster onset of action and longer duration of pain relief than oral morphine.

SPINAL ADMINISTRATION

Since spinal opioid analgesia was introduced in the late 1970s, its use has grown dramatically. It has been used in the intraoperative and postoperative settings, for obstetric analgesia, and for chronic pain of malignant and nonmalignant origin (Cousins and Mather 1984). The opioids, generally morphine and related compounds, are given through either epidural or intrathecal routes. Spinal opioids may be given by intermittent injection through reservoir devices or by continuous infusion through implantable and external pumps.

Spinal opioids offer potential advantages over systemic administration of opioids because lower doses produce longer pain relief. For example, 5 mg of morphine given epidurally provides analgesia for 12 to 18 hours. Disadvantages of the spinal route include more difficult drug delivery and a longer onset of action time. Spinal morphine causes satisfactory

analgesia after 30 to 60 minutes, compared to 5 to 10 minutes for IV morphine (Payne 1987b).

Much has been learned during the last decade about the pharmacology of opioids given by the spinal routes. A sizable proportion of drug in-
jected at the lumbar level intrathecally will ascend in the cerebrospinal
fluid (CSF) (fig. 7.2). The same occurs to that fraction of an epidural dose
that crosses the dura. After intrathecal injection, the less fat-soluble
drugs, such as morphine, will remain longer in the CSF and a higher proportion will be free to travel rostrally. With epidural use, drugs of low fat
solubility are subject to less vascular absorption and a larger fraction is
left to cross the dura. With epidural injections, concentrations of opioids

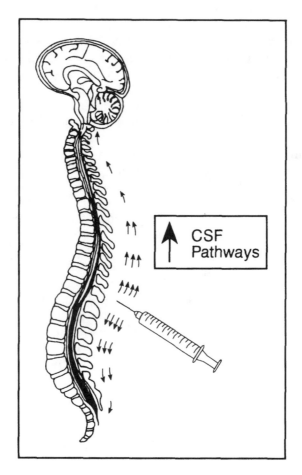

Figure 7.2. The rostral ascent of opioids administered by the spinal route

in plasma can be substantial and may contribute to supraspinal analgesia in a fashion similar to that of conventional parenteral injections.

The present evidence suggests that the analgesic action of spinal opioids comes from a direct action with specific receptors in the spinal cord as well as from a supraspinal effect through blood-borne drug. The duration of analgesia is limited by the life span of the occupied opioid receptors at both spinal and cerebral levels. As noted previously, small doses of epidural morphine can produce long periods of analgesia.

It seems that there is a cross-tolerance between systemic and spinally administered opioids and that tolerance to spinal opioids may develop rapidly. Tolerance, in fact, may be a major factor limiting the effectiveness of spinal opioid analgesia, although Sallerin-Caute et al. (1998) reported that moderate increases in opioid doses did not limit the patient's ability to obtain adequate pain control.

Indications for spinal administration of opioids are still being defined. This route may be particularly helpful to patients with severe bilateral or midline opioid-sensitive pain below the level of the umbilicus, who cannot obtain adequate pain relief with systemic opioids because of dose-limiting side effects. Sacral bone metastasis and lumbosacral plexus involvement with tumor, often seen in patients with genitourinary and colon cancers, are a frequent cause of this type of pain (Payne 1987b, 1989a). In addition, good results have been reported in patients whose oral intake of morphine was at or below the median four-hour requirement of 20 mg. Poor pain control, however, has followed spinal opioid use for pain that was poorly sensitive to systemic opioids (Editorial 1986a). Therefore, the spinal administration of opioids may be useful for patients with opioid-sensitive pain that cannot be managed by conventional routes (table 7.4).

Epidural or intrathecal administration of morphine produces CSF concentrations one or two times greater than those obtained by the systemic route and is associated with significant levels of drug in plasma. Thus, blood-borne drug delivery to the brain, combined with rostral CSF redistribution of drug, may cause unwanted supraspinal side effects, such as respiratory depression, pruritus, urinary retention, and nausea and vomiting.

TABLE 7.4   The Indications for Spinal Administration of Opioids

---

Opioid-sensitive pain not managed by conventional routes due to dose-limiting side effects
Severe bilateral or midline pain below the level of the umbilicus
Pelvic pain due to sacral bone metastasis or lumbosacral plexus involvement with tumor

---

Sources: Editorial (1986a); Payne (1987b, 1989a).

The most serious complication of the spinal administration of opioids is respiratory depression, which may occur early (1 to 2 hours) or late (6 to 24 hours). Early respiratory depression is related to systemic absorption of the drug and its supraspinal effect, whereas late respiratory depression is caused by rostral drug flow in the CSF. A 4 to 7 percent incidence of respiratory depression has been reported after intrathecal morphine. However, fatal respiratory depression has not been associated with the chronic use of opioids by the spinal route.

Certain factors that predispose to respiratory depression after the use of spinal opioids have been identified (Payne 1987b, 1989a):

- advanced age;
- the use of large doses of low fat-soluble drugs, such as morphine;
- lack of systemic opioid tolerance;
- marked changes in intrathoracic pressures, such as might occur with end-expiratory ventilation;
- concomitant administration of opioids and other CNS depressants by systemic routes.

Pruritus occurs in 0 to 80 percent of patients treated with spinal opioids. The characteristics of pruritus are as follows:

- it occurs after acute and chronic administration and is not dose dependent;
- it occurs regardless of the spinal route (i.e., epidural or intrathecal);
- it usually continues for the duration of analgesia;
- it is not segmental, generally occurring on the face and palate;
- it is not related to the preservatives in the drug solution;
- it is not blocked by histamine and may be worsened by coadministration of steroids;
- it occurs more commonly after the administration of systemic or spinal opioids than after the spinal administration of local anesthetics;
- it may be reversed with naloxone;
- it may be severe enough to limit therapy.

The mechanism of spinal opioid-induced pruritus is unknown.

Urinary retention requiring bladder catheterization is seen in 0.3 to 90 percent of patients treated with spinal opioids. Approximately 70 percent of these cases occurred in elderly males. Urinary retention has been reported with low doses, such as 3 to 4 mg epidural, and can last as long as 18 hours after the administration of spinal opioids. The mechanism of this side effect is unknown, but it may involve a direct effect of opioids on the spinal cord to decrease parasympathetic tone to the bladder.

Nausea and vomiting occur in 15 to 75 percent of postoperative, obstetric, and cancer patients treated with spinal opioids. This complication may occur within 10 to 70 minutes after as little as 1 to 2 mg of intrathecal morphine. However, tolerance to this side effect may develop rapidly.

Minimization of the supraspinal component of the above-noted side effects that are related to rostral CSF redistribution of drug may occur with the use of drugs such as methadone and fentanyl. These drugs are more fat soluble and are rapidly cleared from the CSF before rostral ascent to the brainstem.

Two papers are representative of the medical literature on the use of spinal opioids to control cancer pain not relieved by conventional systemic opioid administration. DuPen et al. (1987) treated 55 cancer patients with metastatic disease and intractable pain; they used an exteriorized epidural catheter for the self-administration of morphine. No catheter infections were found during 3,891 catheter-days of use, and only 18 minor side effects (mostly nausea and vomiting) were noted. No respiratory depression was observed. Hospitalization for pain control was decreased by 90 percent.

Penn and Paice (1987) used intrathecal morphine delivered by implanted continuous infusion or programmable devices to manage uncontrolled pain in 35 cancer patients. Twenty-eight (80%) of the patients experienced excellent or good pain relief. Side effects were rare.

A note of caution on the use of spinal opioids was sounded by Devulder et al. (1994). Although a majority (76%) of the 33 cancer patients they treated with intrathecal morphine obtained good pain control, the complication rate was unusually high. Three patients developed bacterial meningitis, which was attributed to accidental disconnection in the external tubing of the pump system. In addition, catheter obstruction occurred in 4 patients, CSF leakage in 3 patients, and postoperative hemorrhage in 1 patient. Because of these complications, the authors advocated the use of intrathecal morphine, if possible, only as a last resort.

Although the use of spinal opioids for pain control represents advancing technology, many questions need to be answered regarding optimal drug use (including dosage and pharmacology), understanding and managing tolerance, and the exact role of this treatment modality in clinical practice. A report by Hogan et al. (1991) placed in perspective the current role of spinal opioids in the management of chronic cancer pain. By aggressively using systemic opioids, they administered epidural morphine to only 15 of 1,205 patients (1.2%); to achieve successful analgesia, bupivacaine had to be added in half the cases. Complications occurred in 11 of these 16 patients. The investigators concluded that spinal opioids are indicated in only a few selected patients.

Ultimately, because of the invasive nature of drug administration via the spinal route and the associated costs (Seamans, Wong, and Wilson 2000) to the patient and family, prospective clinical trials must be performed to compare the effectiveness of spinal opioids to those of current conventional routes.

Transdermal Administration

The use of the transdermal route for drug delivery is not new. In fact, nitroglycerin, clondine, and scopolamine have been used in this manner. Physiologically, the skin serves as a shield to protect the body from the invasion of microorganisms, viruses, and toxic chemicals and to prevent the loss of important vital materials, such as water, from the body. The skin is relatively impermeable to most substances, with the stratum corneum, a layer of skin, being the principal barrier. This impermeability is more passive than active and is closely connected with a drug's minimal ability to diffuse through the intercellular lipid phase of the stratum corneum.

The Transdermal Therapeutic System (TTS) (ALZA Corporation, Palo Alto, California) is one such transdermal system of drug delivery. The TTS consists of an outer backing membrane in contact with the drug reservoir, a drug reservoir containing the active substance, a microporous membrane of specific permeability, a pressure-sensitive adhesive layer that keeps the system on the skin while offering minimal resistance to drug transport, and a protective film, which the patient removes from the system before application (fig. 7.3). The inclusion of a rate-controlling membrane provides an opportunity to diminish fluctuations in drug levels, thereby reducing the potential for exposure to subtherapeutic or toxic serum concentrations.

The TTS was originally developed to test the use of transdermal scopolamine to prevent or relieve travel sickness and nausea. Scopolamine had

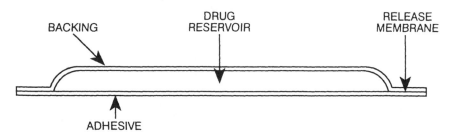

Figure 7.3. A transdermal therapeutic system for the release of fentanyl

long been known to be active against this problem but, because of its marked side effects, it had been used infrequently in conventional dosage forms. Clinical studies with TTS (scopolamine) for motion sickness demonstrated that the release of scopolamine from the system had the desired therapeutic effect without eliciting the bothersome side effects associated with the other forms of dosage. Shortly after the application of TTS, the drug (scopolamine) is released. It saturates the binding sites in the skin. Thereafter, a continuous controlled release of the drug occurs for up to 72 hours. Scopolamine travels via the circulatory system to the target site. After the system is removed from the skin, the drug concentration in the systemic circulation falls to an ineffective level (Heilmann 1978).

Advantages of transdermal drug administration include a high degree of patient acceptability of the noninvasive technique; reduced variations in serum concentrations of the drug, leading to improvement in response and minimization of adverse effects; improved patient compliance as a result of longer dosing intervals and less frequent administration; elimination of gastrointestinal absorption problems related to oral dosing; reduction of drug metabolism because the liver is initially bypassed; and the use of drugs with short biologic half-lives.

Fentanyl citrate is a synthetic opioid analgesic, approximately 75 times more potent than morphine, which is used primarily for sedation in the perioperative setting or for analgesia during dental surgery. Physicochemical characteristics of fentanyl, such as high potency, skin compatibility, low molecular weight, and appropriate solubility, make it suitable for rate-controlled transdermal delivery. Fentanyl is eliminated from the body predominantly by biotransformation in the liver. Studies of fentanyl given by continuous IV infusion for postoperative analgesia suggest that the dosage of approximately 100 µg/hour is effective and well tolerated in adults (Plezia et al. 1989).

Two studies (Caplan et al. 1989; Plezia et al. 1989) evaluated TTS (fentanyl) in the postoperative setting. Plezia et al. (1989) studied eight patients, who had undergone orthopedic surgery, for 24 hours postoperatively. Two hours before surgery, the TTS (fentanyl) was applied to each patient's upper anterior chest wall, and it remained in place for 24 hours. The nominal delivery rate of the system was 75 µg/hour. Serum samples were obtained over a 72-hour period for pharmacokinetic study in five patients. Transdermal administration of fentanyl was very well tolerated in this group of patients. Adverse reactions were minimal. Pharmacokinetic analysis suggested continuous delivery of the drug after a two-hour lag period, with prolonged elimination. Prolongation of fentanyl elimination resulted from the formation of a deposit of the drug in the fatty skin tissue underneath the transdermal system. After removal of the device, drug diffused away from the site at a gradually declining rate, giving the appearance of prolonged elimination. This phenomenon was responsible for the lag time from the application of the transdermal system to the appearance of drug in circulation. In that setting, the transdermal administration of fentanyl seemed to be a viable alternative to conventional routes of opioid administration and warranted further investigation.

In a larger, double-blind, placebo-controlled study, Caplan et al. (1989) evaluated the safety and efficacy of transdermal fentanyl for the management of postoperative pain in 42 healthy adult patients undergoing major shoulder surgery. The TTS (fentanyl) was used, and, as with the previous study, fentanyl was delivered at a rate of 75 μg/hour. TTS (fentanyl) was applied to the skin immediately before surgery and was worn for 24 hours. Patients in the fentanyl group required significantly less morphine than did those in the placebo group during the 24-hour period when the systems were in place and during the first 12 hours after removal. The incidence of vomiting and lowered respiratory rate, however, was higher. As noted by the authors, this slow decline in serum fentanyl levels may offer a potential advantage in that the transition to other forms of pain management may occur without an abrupt loss of analgesia. The investigators concluded that transdermal fentanyl seems to be safe and effective after orthopedic surgery in healthy adult patients and that transdermal delivery of fentanyl produces an agreeable, constant quality of pain control that is superior to conventional therapy with IM morphine.

In 1989, Miser et al. reported their experience in using TTS delivery to treat five cancer patients with transdermal fentanyl. Patients were initially begun on a continuous IV infusion of fentanyl to achieve satisfactory pain control. After this endpoint was reached, TTS (fentanyl) patches were applied to the chest wall, back, or upper arm and were routinely changed every 24 hours, as preclinical testing with these systems had demonstrated constant drug delivery for this period. Also, skin sites were rotated with each application. The TTS delivered drugs at 25, 50, or 100 μg/hour. The five patients, who were aged 16 to 68 years old, had a history of poor pain control due to an inability to take oral analgesics or because these drugs were ineffective in controlling pain. Overall, the patients experienced satisfactory pain relief for periods of 3 to 156 days (mean of 145 days) using continuous transdermal delivery of fentanyl. Dosages were adjusted to each patient's need and varied from 75 to 350 μg/hour, with a median of 225 μg/hour. No patient developed skin irritation at the site of application. Major clinical difficulties noted in the study included the delay in obtaining steady-state serum concentrations of fentanyl (which led to minor overdosing in two patients) and the prolonged period of continued fentanyl effect after TTS removal. This prolonged effect became an important clinical issue when unrelated medical complications arose suddenly in patients and a more rapid change in opioid level was desired. As noted by the authors, transdermal delivery of opioid provides an ideal analgesic modality for patients with chronic pain who are in stable clinical condition and who otherwise would have required parenteral opioids. In this study, transdermal fentanyl permitted home care for three of the five patients.

In a larger study, Simmonds et al. (1989) investigated TTS (fentanyl) in 39 patients with various forms of advanced cancer. The opioid treatment was converted to oral morphine and titrated to a stable dose. Conversion was made to TTS, which was applied every three days. Immediate-release morphine was prescribed for breakthrough pain. There were 16 female and 23 male patients, with a median age of 61 years. The median morphine stabilization dosage was 120 mg/day. The median dosage of fentanyl at the start of the study was 50 µg/hour (range of 25 to 225) and the median current or final dosage was 100 µg/hour (range of 25 to 525). More than half of the patients increased their dosage by 50 percent or more while on the study. The patients were able to maintain the TTS patch through a variety of concomitant events, such as surgery for pathologic fracture, herpes zoster infection, and chemotherapy infusions. Thus, the authors suggested, the clinical use and safety of TTS (fentanyl) in this group of cancer patients have been demonstrated. Patient compliance and acceptance are excellent.

Two studies (Ahmedzai and Brooks 1997; Payne et al. 1998) compared transdermal fentanyl to oral controlled-release morphine. Ahmedzai and Brooks (1997) studied 202 cancer patients who required opioid analgesia. Fifty-five percent of these patients were men and the mean age was 61.5 years, with a range of 18 to 89 years. In this randomized, cross-over study, patients received either transdermal fentanyl or controlled-release morphine for 15 days, followed immediately by the other treatment for 15 additional days. Fentanyl was associated with significantly less constipation and less daytime drowsiness but greater sleep disturbance and shorter sleep duration than morphine. There was no significant difference in quality of life between the two treatment groups. Of those patients able to express a preference, significantly more preferred TTS (fentanyl). The authors concluded that, in this study, transdermal fentanyl provided pain relief that was acceptable to cancer patients and was associated with less constipation and sedation than controlled-release morphine.

In a related investigation, Payne et al. (1998) assessed quality of life in 504 cancer patients who received controlled-release oral morphine and transdermal fentanyl for cancer pain. Overall, patient demographics in the two treatment groups were similar, except that patients in the transdermal fentanyl group were significantly older than patients in the oral morphine group. The majority of patients in both treatment groups had advanced cancer. The mean dose of transdermal fentanyl was 84.35 µg/hour and the median dose was 75 µg/hour, whereas the mean 24-hour dose of controlled-release oral morphine was 194.95 mg and the median dose was 120 mg. Patients who received transdermal fentanyl were more satisfied overall with their pain medication than those who received controlled-release oral morphine. Fentanyl patients experienced a significantly lower frequency and impact of pain medication side effects even though they were significantly older than patients in the morphine group. Measures of pain intensity, sleep adequacy, and symptoms showed no significant differences between treatment groups. These data suggest, as reported by the authors, that patients are more satisfied with transdermal fentanyl than with controlled-release oral morphine. A lower frequency and reduced impact of side effects with transdermal fentanyl may be one reason, the authors speculated, why cancer patients who receive fentanyl are more satisfied with their pain management.

Payne (1992) provided the following guidelines for the use of transdermal fentanyl:

- Patients with stable baseline pain and minimal incident pain are good candidates for this route of administration because frequent dose adjustments are difficult to achieve with transdermal fentanyl. It is usually necessary to obtain adequate baseline pain control with conventional opioid dosing before initiating treatment with transdermal fentanyl.
- Because of the unique pharmacokinetics of fentanyl delivered transdermally, the liberal use of immediate-release analgesics for rescue dosing is often necessary, especially when therapy is being started or when the dosage is being adjusted. The average 72-hour rescue dose of analgesics is used to calculate dose changes of transdermal fentanyl at the time of the next patch application.
- Rotate skin sites to minimize variations in blood level due to the excess accumulation of SC deposits of fentanyl. Warn patients about poor skin adhesion resulting from sweating and hair growth.
- Because of the increased risks of side effects associated with the use of long-acting opioids, transdermal fentanyl should not be routinely administered with controlled- release morphine, methadone, or levorphanol.

To aid in the calculation of the dosage of transdermal fentanyl, Johanson (1992) and Enck (1995) recommended the following approximate equivalencies in the chronic, steady state:

- 25 μg/hour patch = 10 mg oral morphine every 4 hours or 60 mg/ 24 hour oral morphine
- 50 μg/hour patch = 20 mg oral morphine every 4 hours or 120 mg/ 24 hour oral morphine
- 75 μg/hour patch = 30 mg oral morphine every 4 hours or 180 mg/ 24 hour oral morphine
- 100 μg/hour patch = 40 mg oral morphine every 4 hours or 240 mg/24 hour oral morphine

The success of the TTS (fentanyl) model is directly related to the permeability of fentanyl across the skin barrier. The same is not true for morphine. Using an animal model, Sugibayashi, Sakanoue, and Morimoto (1989) studied the role of skin penetration enhancers added to morphine hydrochloride. They found that the addition of azone and N-methyl-2 pyrrolidone to a morphine solution significantly enhanced the skin permeation of morphine. Much more preclinical research is needed in this area before topical morphine can be clinically tested with patients.

Summary

Oral morphine is the drug of choice for chronic severe pain. In most cases, it can be given by this route until death. Administered as an immediate-release preparation at four-hour intervals, oral morphine produces analgesia within 60 minutes, with a peak effect at 1.5 to 2.0 hours and a four-to seven-hour duration. Because of wide individual variation in the metabolism of morphine, there is a broad therapeutic dose range for good pain control. The oral:parenteral potency in chronic pain is 2–3:1; thus, the usual starting dose in an opioid-naive patient is 20 to 30 mg every four hours. According to pharmacokinetic studies, older patients require smaller doses of morphine for pain control than do younger patients. Use four-hour dosing of oral morphine for initial pain stabilization as well as for breakthrough pain when long-acting preparations are employed.

As evidenced by a study from the United Kingdom (White et al. 1991), there is considerable confusion and misperception concerning the use of controlled-release morphine such as MS Contin. This, in turn, has led to its misuse, especially in regard to the frequency of administration and escalation of the dosage. Multiple clinical studies have demonstrated that controlled-release morphine administered at 12-hour intervals produces pain control equivalent to that of oral morphine given every four hours. Controlled-release oral morphine should be used for maintenance therapy once the patient's morphine requirement is determined; it is inappropriate for use "as needed." When converting patients from immediate-release oral morphine preparations to the controlled-release formulation, use a potency ratio of 1:1. Additional controlled-release oral opioids, such as oxycodone, are available and seem to be as safe and effective as controlled-release morphine.

Continuous parenteral infusions of opioids, regardless of the route, are safe and are associated with low toxicity except in those rare patients requiring more than 4 grams of IV morphine per day in whom seizures may occur because of the excess accumulation of bisulfate preservatives. The continuous SC route offers better quality-of-life satisfaction for the patient than does the IV route.

Continuous parenteral infusions of opioids coupled with patient-controlled analgesia (PCA) bolus for breakthrough pain is highly effective for relieving pain and can be safely administered at home. This PCA technique is most advantageous in managing incident pain.

Using a mucosal membrane route (such as sublingual, buccal, or rectal) to administer opioid analgesics produces a more rapid onset and a longer duration of analgesia. This route is especially useful when the patient is near death and unable to swallow.

Giving opioids via the spinal route is another alternative in providing analgesia. Lower dosages of spinal morphine administered either intrathecally or epidurally produce longer analgesia than do those by conventional routes. Indications for the spinal administration of opioids are still being defined. Many scientific questions remain unanswered regarding the use of spinal opioids to manage chronic cancer pain, including the optimal drug use, tolerance, cost, and the exact role of this treatment modality in clinical practice. Until these answers are provided, conventional routes of administering opioids remain the standard of care except in select patients.

Technology is available to deliver drugs transdermally in a rate-controlled fashion over a long period. Fentanyl, a synthetic opioid analgesic, is 75 times more potent than morphine and can penetrate the skin. Like the controlled-release preparations of morphine, transdermal fentanyl is useful for patients with stable chronic pain and minimal discomfort associated with movement.

Chapter 8

Adjuvant Analgesic Drugs

Drugs added to opioid analgesics to improve the control of cancer pain are referred to as either *coanalgesics* (Twycross and Hanks 1984; De Conno 1998) or *adjuvant analgesic drugs* (Foley and Arbit 1989; Payne 1991; Jacox et al. 1994). The scientific rationale for using these drugs is often anecdotal, with few clinical studies in cancer patients with pain. There also appears to be little agreement as to what agents to include in this category. To ensure a uniform approach, I shall use the term *adjuvant analgesic drugs,* and I include in this group anticonvulsants, phenothiazines, antidepressants, antihistamines, steroids, and antibiotics.

Anticonvulsants

Anticonvulsants, such as phenytoin and carbamazepine, are well-known effective drugs for the management of pain in chronic neuralgias (such as trigeminal neuralgia, postherpetic neuralgia, glossopharyngeal neuralgia, and posttraumatic neuralgias). With cancer pain, carbamazepine is useful in managing the acute, shocklike neuralgic pain in the cranial and cervical distribution caused by infiltration by the tumor or surgical injury to the nerve. It also is effective for patients with involvement of the lumbosacral plexus (Payne 1991). In one of the few studies done in cancer patients, phenytoin was compared with buprenorphine alone and a combination of phenytoin and buprenorphine in 25 patients with cancer pain. Good or moderate pain relief was obtained in more than 60 percent of the patients (McQuay et al. 1995). In two randomized, controlled trials, the anticonvulsant gabapentin was reported to be effective in relieving the pain of diabetic peripheral neuropathy (Backonja et al. 1998) and postherpetic neuralgia (Rowbotham et al. 1998).

Phenothiazines

The phenothiazines, with the possible exception of methotrimepra-zine, play a minimal role in the management of cancer pain. Methotri-meprazine, available only in the parenteral form, exhibits analgesic properties and is useful in special circumstances, such as opioid toler-ance or the need to avoid the constipating effects of opioids while main-taining analgesia. The combination of fluphenazine and a tricyclic anti-depressant may prove useful for the management of nerve injury pain (Payne 1991), but, as in other areas, agreement is not uniform (Hanks 1984). Combining a phenothiazine, such as prochlorperazine, and an opioid analgesic heightens only sedation and not pain control. Because of this and other enhancements of side effects, the routine use of a phenothiazine as an antiemetic combined with an opioid is strongly con-demned.

Antidepressants

Tricyclic antidepressants are one group of drugs that most agree play a role in pain management. Their direct analgesic effects are provided by blocking of the reuptake of serotonin and norepinephrine at the central nervous system synapses. Another mechanism of action may relate to the emotional component of pain perception. In a review, Magni, Conlon, and Arsie (1987) concluded that the tricyclic antidepressants seem to be useful in reducing cancer pain that may or may not be associated with de-pressive symptoms. The dosage is similar to that used in the treatment of depression. Furthermore, the authors suggested that, when the tricyclics are used concurrently with opioids, a dose reduction in the opioid anal-gesics and a potentiation of analgesia are possible. Others (Foley and Ar-bit 1989; Payne 1991) thought that analgesic effects are more evident at lower doses (e.g., 10 to 150 mg daily for amitriptyline) than are the anti-depressant effects. In one of the few controlled clinical trials, amitripty-line demonstrated significant analgesia in the management of posther-petic neuralgia as compared to placebo (Watson et al. 1982). Controlled trials demonstrated that several of the newer antidepressants, such as the selective serotonin reuptake inhibitor (SSRI) paroxetine, have analgesic effect. Very few of the other newer antidepressants have been studied, and evidence of pain relief is limited to favorable anecdotes (Portenoy 1998).

Antihistamines

Of the antihistamines, hydroxyzine is the most frequently used in clinical practice. It may produce additive analgesia, in doses of 25 to 100 mg daily, when combined with opioids (Payne 1991; Jacox et al. 1994).

Steroids

Steroids are another group of drug that may act as adjuvant analgesic agents in certain clinical circumstances, such as spinal cord compression due to tumor, brain metastases, and compression or infiltration of nerve by tumor. In these instances, steroids offer pain relief by decreasing the soft tissue swelling in the area of the tumor focus (Jacox et al. 1994). Dexa methasone seems to be the steroid of choice for these clinical situations (Twycross and Hanks 1984). Claims for the use of steroids, for example, in patients with soft tissue tumor infiltration and hepatomegaly (Hanks and Justins 1992) are poorly substantiated.

Antibiotics

Antibiotics may be useful in certain clinical circumstances, such as acute infection associated with malignant ulceration (Bruera and Mac-Donald 1986) and cellulitis (Hanks and Justins 1992). Bruera and Mac-Donald (1986) observed seven patients with locally advanced head and neck carcinoma who had a sudden increase in their pain that improved with antibiotics. All of these patients had large ulcerated masses surrounded by chronic swelling and erythema before the onset of the severe pain. Significant relief from pain was obtained in all patients within three days of starting the antibiotic therapy. The authors suggested that acute local infection is probably a frequent event and the clinician should suspect it in patients with head and neck cancers who show a rapidly changing pattern of pain. Furthermore, signs of local infection as well as fever and leukocytosis may be absent, and a therapeutic trial of antibiotics may be necessary in these cases.

Amphetamines

There is a resurgence of interest in the use of amphetamines as adjuvant analgesic agents in the management of chronic cancer pain. In 1944 Ivy et al. were the first to demonstrate that dextroamphetamine enhanced the analgesic effect of morphine in 450 patients with acute postoperative pain (Forrest et al. 1977). The investigators found, in this double-blind, single-dose study, that analgesia was augmented with the combination of drugs. Dextroamphetamine, 5 mg, in conjunction with a certain dose of morphine provided pain relief equivalent to that obtained with one and one-half times that dose of morphine taken alone. Adding dextroamphetamine, 10 mg, to morphine has the analgesic effect of approximately twice that dose of morphine alone. The Forrest et al. (1977) study, however, was in the acute pain noncancer setting.

In 1982, Joshi et al. reported their experience with amphetamines in terminally ill cancer patients. Nineteen patients were given dextroamphetamine at a starting dose of 2.5 mg every six hours. In this noncontrolled study, 16 patients were evaluable for response. Improvements, as recorded by two physician observers, were noted in mood (87%), activity level (75%), pain (70%), and appetite (43%). In a subsequent controlled clinical study with a double-blind, cross-over design, Bruera et al. (1986a) compared a mild amphetamine, mazindol, with a placebo to determine its effectiveness for symptom control in 30 terminally ill cancer patients. The authors reported that mazindol was associated with severe toxicity in the form of delirium (2 patients) that required the discontinuation of the treatment. The use of mazindol, as employed in this study, did not significantly improve comfort in any of the patients. However, the data suggested that the use of mazindol decreased the intensity of the pain and the consumption of oral analgesics. Patients enrolled in this study had only mild or moderate pain.

In 1987, this same group (Bruera et al. 1987d) evaluated the adjuvant analgesic properties of methylphenidate in 32 patients with advanced cancer. All patients were receiving opioids on a regular basis and were treated with methylphenidate (10 mg orally with breakfast and 5 mg orally with lunch) for three days versus placebo in a randomized double-blind, cross-over study. In the 28 evaluable patients, methylphenidate potentiated the analgesic effects of the opioids, decreased drowsiness, and significantly increased the level of patient activity. After the study was completed, the investigator and the patient chose methylphenidate blindly as a more useful drug in 23 cases (82%) and 20 cases (71%), respectively. Severe toxicity was not observed. Although low-dose methylphenidate combined with opioid analgesics may have a role in managing severe cancer pain, the authors cautioned that amphetamines may enhance mental abnormalities in this situation. Therefore, until future study, Bruera et al. (1987d) did not recommend the more general use of methylphenidate for improving the comfort of terminally ill patients. However, based on the studies by Bruera et al. (1987d) and Joshi et al. (1982), the expert panel that developed the *Clinical Practice Guideline for the Management of Cancer Pain* (Jacox et al. 1994) recommended the use of dextroamphetamine and methylphenidate to improve opioid analgesia and decrease sedation. Clearly, more clinical research is necessary to determine the role of psychostimulants in pain management.

Butyrophenones

The butyrophenone haloperidol potentiates morphine analgesia in animals; however, there are few clinical data to support these effects in humans. In a review of the literature, Hanks (1984) was unable to substantiate an opioid-sparing effect of haloperidol and did not advocate its use.

Finally, several groups of drug should be avoided in the management of chronic cancer pain: the benzodiazepines, sedative-hypnotics such as the barbiturates, canabinoids, and cocaine (Payne 1991; Jacox et al. 1994).

Summary

Despite the paucity of sound clinical studies of patients with cancer pain, adjuvant analgesics still play an important role in the management of pain. The anticonvulsants, such as carbamazepine and gabapentin, are helpful in managing neuropathic pain, as are the tricyclic antidepressants, especially amitriptyline. The routine use of a phenothiazine as an antiemetic enhances only sedation and not pain control and therefore is inappropriate. Steroids, mainly dexamethasone, are indicated in cases of the involvement or compression of the nervous system by the tumor. Antibiotics may improve pain control in patients with acute local infections, as occurs in patients with advanced head and neck cancer. Despite encouraging preliminary results, the routine use of amphetamines as adjuvant therapy is still being debated.

Chapter 9

Complications of Pharmacologic Therapy

Although chronic pain may be effectively controlled with a wide variety of pharmacologic agents, this is often associated with untoward side effects. In some cases, these side effects become so burdensome that they interfere with the goal of patient comfort. Therefore, not only is the understanding of pharmacologic intervention important in pain control strategies but also an appreciation of the side effects and how they are managed is critical to good patient care.

Opioids

Certain risks expose the patient to a greater likelihood of having a drug-related complication. Age is a major factor. Older patients are more sensitive to opioids and their side effects than are younger patients. Prior treatment with opioids and the route of administration are also important. For example, sublingual, buccal, and rectal administration of morphine has fewer side effects than the oral route. The presence of underlying medical problems, especially pulmonary disease, may enhance untoward reactions to pain-management therapies. Patients with pulmonary dysfunction are at greater risk for developing opioid-induced respiratory depression than are patients with normal lung function. Finally, it is worth noting that a true allergy to morphine is rare (Levy 1996).

In 1987, Ventafridda et al. reported their two-year experience using the World Health Organization (WHO) three-step treatment for cancer pain. In brief, this analgesia ladder starts with nonopioids, such as aspirin, acetaminophen, and other nonsteroidal anti-inflammatory drugs (NSAIDs). As the pain progresses, the next step is the use of weak opioids (codeine, for example). The final step, if the pain persists, is the use of the strong opioids (i.e., morphine and related compounds). Adjuvant analgesics may be used as well.

TABLE 9.1 The Frequency of Side Effects Associated with the WHO Analgesia Ladder

Side Effect	Frequency (%)
Dry mouth	39
Drowsiness	38
Constipation	35
Sweating	23
Nausea/vomiting	22
Stomach ache	17
Agitation	16
Itching	10
Blood loss	6
None	24

Source: Ventafridda et al. (1987).

The investigators calculated the percentage of days on which side effects were present during a two-month follow-up of patients treated. Over the entire span of the three-step treatment, the most frequent side effects were dry mouth, drowsiness, constipation, sweating, and nausea/vomiting (table 9.1).

Not surprisingly, there were no side effects in more patients given nonopioids than in those given strong opioids (39% versus 21%). More dry mouth, drowsiness, constipation, and sweating were reported by the patients treated with the strong opioids, predominantly morphine, than by patients given either nonopioids or weak opioids.

DRY MOUTH

Although the study by Ventafridda et al. (1987) identified dry mouth as the most frequent side effect of treatment using the WHO analgesia ladder, it is difficult to attribute this complication to a single drug because most patients were taking multiple drugs. Therefore, a study by White et al. (1989) is helpful in identifying a cause for this complication. These investigators studied the prevalence of dryness of the mouth in patients with cancer to determine if it was related to the use of morphine. All patients admitted to the Continuing Care Unit of Royal Marsden Hospital, in London, during an eight-week period were entered into the study except those who had other reasons for having a dry mouth (such as those receiving radiation therapy, surgery, chemotherapy, or the like). Data were obtained from 199 patients. One hundred thirty-one patients were using opioid analgesics, and 67 were taking morphine. One hundred nineteen of 199 patients (57%) reported dryness of the mouth at some time during the course of treatment; of these 119, 42 (37%) had a dry mouth most or all of the time. There was no significant correlation between the severity of the mouth dryness and sex, age, primary diagnosis, reason for admission, the wearing of dentures, oral candidiasis, or smoking. Analysis showed a highly significant association between the use of morphine and dryness of the mouth. When the results were controlled for concurrent treatment, patients receiving morphine were approximately four times more likely to have dry mouth of any severity than were patients taking weak opioids, nonopioids, or no analgesics.

The mechanisms for the adverse effect of morphine were unclear. As noted by the authors, recognition of this side effect is important, and careful attention should be paid to oral comfort and hygiene. A simple measure, such as frequent sips of cool drinks or sucking on ice cubes, may help relieve this dry mouth (O'Neill and Fallon 1997).

RESPIRATORY DEPRESSION

In a review of analgesic drug therapy for chronic cancer pain, Foley and Inturrisi (1987) suggested that the most common side effects of opioid analgesics are sedation, nausea and vomiting, constipation, and respiratory depression. With the exception of respiratory depression, these are similar to those reported by Ventafridda et al. (1987) (table 9.2).

Respiratory depression is potentially the most serious side effect of opioid therapy. Morphine and related drugs act on brainstem respiratory centers to produce dose-dependent respiratory depression. Therapeutic doses of morphine may depress all phases of respiration. However, as carbon dioxide accumulates, it stimulates the respiratory centers, resulting in a compensatory increase in respiratory rate, which, in turn, hides the degree of respiratory depression. At equivalent doses, all the morphine-related drugs produce the same degree of respiratory depression. For

TABLE 9.2   The Clinically Important Side Effects of Opioids

CNS-Related Side Effects	Non-CNS-Related Side Effects
Drowsiness/sedation	Dry mouth
Nausea/vomiting	Constipation
Agitation, nightmares, anxiety, euphoria, dysphoria, depression, paranoia, hallucinations	Sweating Itching Urinary retention
Respiratory depression	

Sources: Foley and Inturrisi (1987); Ventafridda et al. (1987); Medical Letter (1989a); O'Neill and Fallon (1997).

Note: Side effects are listed in decreasing order of frequency.

these reasons, Foley and Inturrisi (1987) suggested that patients with impaired respiratory function or bronchial asthma are at greater risk for experiencing clinically significant respiratory depression in response to the usual dosages of these drugs.

Respiratory depression usually occurs with the acute administration of morphine to an opioid-naive patient and is often accompanied by other signs of central nervous system (CNS) depression, such as sedation and confusion. A tolerance of the effect develops rapidly with repeated administration of the drug, thus typically allowing opioid analgesics to be used in the management of chronic pain without significant risk of respiratory depression. As noted by Clark and Edwards (1999), patients with gastrointestinal motility disorders, such as gastroparesis, may be at high risk for respiratory depression from orally administered opioids due to altered absorption kinetics.

If respiratory depression occurs, it may be reversed by the administration of the specific opioid antagonist naloxone. For patients being treated with opioids chronically who develop respiratory depression, naloxone diluted 1:10 should be titrated carefully to prevent the precipitation of severe withdrawal symptoms (Foley and Inturrisi 1987).

The major effect of the opioids on the CNS is sedation or drowsiness. Because of an additive effect, clinicians must exercise care in the use of other CNS depressants, such as alcohol, barbiturates, and benzodiazepines in combination with opioids. A tolerance of sedation usually develops within the first several days of chronic administration of opioids. Indeed, Vainio et al. (1995) studied driving function in 24 cancer patients taking a mean dose of 209 mg/day of oral morphine. They found that the long-term use of oral morphine only slightly impaired the ability of these patients to drive, again demonstrating the occurrence of tolerance to opioid-induced sedation.

Nausea and Vomiting

Opioid analgesics produce nausea and vomiting by acting on the medullary chemoreceptor trigger zone. The tendency of these drugs to cause nausea and vomiting varies from patient to patient, so there may be some advantage in changing opioids for patients experiencing this side effect. Alternatively, antiemetics may be combined with the opioid. However, the choice of antiemetics is important because drugs, such as the phenothiazines, may only enhance opioid-induced sedation.

Other Side Effects on the Central Nervous System

Other, less frequent side effects on the CNS include nightmares, anxiety, agitation, euphoria, dysphoria, depression, paranoia, and hallucinations. These generally occur with high doses of opioids, with the possible exception of meperidine and methadone (*Medical Letter* 1989a). Accumulation of the metabolite normeperidine in patients treated chronically with meperidine causes excitation of the CNS. For this reason, this drug is not recommended for use in the management of chronic cancer pain. Clinicians must also take care when using methadone. Because of its long half-life (15 to 30 hours), methadone in chronic dosing can lead to drug accumulation, which can lead to oversedation and, rarely, coma.

Constipation

Constipation is a common side effect of opioid analgesics. These drugs act at multiple sites throughout the gastrointestinal tract and spinal cord to cause a decrease in intestinal secretions and peristalsis. The net effect is constipation. A tolerance of the smooth muscle effects of opioids develops very slowly, so constipation persists when these drugs are used for chronic pain. The route of opioid administration may influence the incidence of constipation. Clinical trials have consistently shown that there is less constipation in patients treated with transdermal fentanyl than with patients receiving oral morphine (Haazen et al. 1999). When opioids are started, the clinician should give careful attention to managing this side effect. A measure such as increasing ambulation and fluid intake, beginning a diet high in fiber, or trying a bulk laxative should be initiated. The daily administration of a stool softener is also helpful. In addition, low-dose methylnaltrexone (Yuan et al. 2000) and oral erythromycin (Clark and Edwards 1999) may have some clinical usefulness in managing opioid-induced constipation. Further clinical research on the role of these drugs in treating opioid-induced constipation is needed.

Retention of Urine

Another side effect of the opioid analgesics is bladder spasm and an increase in smooth muscle sphincter tone leading to urinary retention. This is most common in older patients and is transient. The itching and sweating associated with opioids is most likely related to histamine release.

Addiction

Fear of addiction to opioid analgesics remains a major impediment to good pain control. This perception is shared by both the patient and caregivers and is further reinforced by the ongoing battle with illicit drug use as highlighted in the news media. Physicians are often reluctant to prescribe opioids until "the last" because of this problem. A survey of 200 Wisconsin physicians by Weissman, Joranson, and Hopwood (1991) found that physicians were more concerned about inducing addiction, tolerance, or respiratory depression than about potentially being investigated for drug diversion.

In a similar fashion, patients are afraid to start treatment with the opioids, often despite the presence of severe uncontrolled pain, because they do not want to be "hooked" on these drugs. Many times the patient's negative perception of opioids is strongly reinforced by family members.

Much of the confusion regarding opioids and addiction is related to a poor understanding of terminology, specifically, *tolerance, physical dependence,* and *psychological dependence* or *addiction. Tolerance* occurs when, after repeated administrations of a drug, a larger dose must be given to obtain the effects observed with the original dose. On the other hand, *physical dependence* refers to an altered physiologic state produced by the repeated administration of a drug to the extent that a sudden cessation of the drug results in withdrawal symptoms. Finally, *psychological dependence* or *addiction* is a behavioral pattern of drug use characterized by overwhelming involvement with the use of the drug and the securing of its supply and a high tendency to relapse after withdrawal (Jaffe 1985).

Tolerance. Tolerance, or the need for escalating opioid doses to maintain adequate analgesia, seems to develop in all patients receiving opioids chronically. The rate of development of this phenomenon, however, varies greatly among cancer patients. Data from animals show that tolerance to morphine occurs in rodents within 24 hours, reaching a maximum within one week. This suggests that more than one week of patient exposure to this drug may lead to tolerance (Chapman and Hill 1989).

The first indication of tolerance is the patient's complaint that the duration of analgesia is decreased from that of the initial administration. Frequently, the patient is labeled as a "clock watcher," a sign that is often viewed by caregivers as an early sign of addiction.

Studies indicate that there are three patterns of drug use in cancer patients:

- rapidly escalating dosages of opioids associated with increasing pain and/or anxiety;
- stable dosages of opioids for long periods (weeks to months) without escalation or reduction of the dosage, and;
- discontinuance of opioid drugs with effective analgesia from cancer therapies or anesthetic or neurosurgical approaches.

These patterns are independent of the route of administering the drug, with progression of painful disease as the overriding factor determining the escalation of the dosage. Although the rate of developing tolerance may vary from patient to patient, a sudden dramatic increase in opioid requirements may well signal a progression of the cancer rather than the development of tolerance.

There appears to be no limit to tolerance. Regardless of the current dosage, dose escalation is appropriate when the goal is effective analgesia. The majority of patients treated by the Supportive Care Program at Memorial Sloan-Kettering Cancer Center required doses in the range of 5 mg to 300 mg of intramuscular morphine equivalents daily. Some patients required very high doses (Foley 1989). Inexperienced physicians may misinterpret these high doses as inappropriate. They undermedicate patients because of their concern for using only standard dosages rather than seeking adequate analgesia as the endpoint.

Of equal importance is the recognition that cross-tolerance is incomplete. Changing patients from one opioid analgesic to another can improve analgesia.

Finally, tolerance of the various side effects of opioids occurs at different rates. Tolerance of respiratory depression develops rapidly, whereas tolerance of constipation develops very slowly. The rapid development of tolerance of the respiratory depressant effects of opioids allows the escalation of dosages in some patients to very high levels.

Physical Dependence. Physical dependence is the pharmacologic effect of opioids. Withdrawal symptoms occur when the drug is stopped. The severity of withdrawal is a function of the duration and dosage of opioid that was discontinued. Patients treated with therapeutic doses of morphine several times a day for one to two weeks will have only mild symptoms that may not be recognized as withdrawal when the drug is stopped. These symptoms may be even less pronounced when the opioid is one that is slowly eliminated, such as methadone (Jaffe 1985).

The onset of withdrawal is heralded by the patient's report of feelings of anxiety, nervousness, irritability, and alternating chills and hot flushes. A prominent withdrawal sign is wetness, including salivation, lacrimation, rhinorrhea, and diaphoresis. Nausea and vomiting, abdominal cramps, insomnia, and, rarely, multifocal myoclonus may occur at the peak intensity of the withdrawal syndrome. The timing of withdrawal is a function of the elimination half-life of the opioid to which the patient has become physically dependent. For example, symptoms will appear within 6 to 12 hours and reach a peak at 24 to 72 hours after the cessation of a short half-life drug such as morphine. With methadone, which has a long half-life, withdrawal symptoms may be delayed for 36 to 48 hours. Even for patients whose pain has been completely relieved by a therapeutic procedure, it is necessary to decrease the opioid dosage slowly to prevent withdrawal symptoms.

The usual daily dose required to prevent withdrawal is equal to one-fourth of the previous daily dose, and it is administered every six hours, or four times per day. This initial withdrawal regimen is administered for two days and then reduced by one-half. This amount is also divided into doses given four times daily for two days. After two days on this dose, the patient can stop the opioid. Thus, a patient who had been receiving 240 mg of morphine per day for pain control would require an initial dose of 60 mg administered in 15 mg doses every six hours (Foley and Inturrisi 1987).

The administration of an opioid antagonist, such as naloxone, to a physically dependent patient immediately precipitates the withdrawal syndrome. Patients being treated with repeated doses of a morphinelike agonist to the point where they are physically dependent may experience an opioid withdrawal reaction when given a mixed agonist-antagonist, like pentazocine. Prior exposure to a morphinelike drug greatly increases a patient's sensitivity to the antagonist component of a mixed agonist-antagonist drug.

Psychological Dependence. Tolerance and physical dependence are predictable pharmacologic effects seen in response to the repeated administration of opioids in both humans and laboratory animals. These effects are distinctly different from the abnormal behavioral patterns seen in some individuals and described by the term *psychological dependence* or *addiction.* Addiction is characterized by a continued craving for opioids as manifested by compulsive drug-seeking behavior and overwhelming involvement in the procurement and use of the drug. The development of addiction is a complex phenomenon in which the type of individual, the reason for drug use, the environment, and the drug play major and, at times, equivalent roles. This concept was well described in the epidemic addiction seen in Vietnam War veterans who rapidly discontinued their heroin use once home, without the use of maintenance programs and with low rates of relapse (Foley 1989).

It is clearly possible for patients taking opioids on a chronic basis, such as those with cancer pain, to be physically dependent without evidence of addiction. As noted by Angell (1982), addiction among patients who receive opioids for pain is exceedingly unlikely, and the incidence is probably no greater than 0.1 percent. Further support for this low addiction rate comes from a study by Chapman and Hill (1989). These investigators studied 26 patients who required opioid analgesics for severe oral mucositis after bone marrow transplantation. Twelve patients self-administered morphine via a patient-controlled analgesia (PCA) system for two weeks. The other 14 patients acted as controls and were given morphine by routine staff-controlled continuous infusion procedures. Self-administering patients used significantly less morphine than the controls and still achieved the same amount of pain control. In addition, the self-administering patients terminated drug use sooner than did the control patients. The investigators concluded that the results support the assumption that self-administration of opioids in a medical setting does not put patients at risk for overmedication or addiction. Finally, Joranson et al. (2000) reported that, despite an increasing trend in the medical use of opioids to treat pain, there did not appear to be a corresponding increase in opioid abuse.

As reported by Hoffman et al. (1991), a special problem is pain management for cancer patients who were abusing opioids before the onset of the cancer. These investigators described the difficulty in pain management due to problems of distinguishing tolerance from disease progression, concurrent methadone maintenance, and drug-seeking behavior. Suggested guidelines for the management of this problem are as follows:

• Provide early psychological help.
• Take complaints of pain at face value and investigated as necessary.
• Set limits (e.g., through a medication contract). This is of critical importance.
• Prescribe medication on a time-contingent basis;
• Continue the maintenance dose of patients on methadone maintenance while their pain is being treated with other opioid agonists.

Nonsteroidal Anti-inflammatory Drugs

The nonsteroidal anti-inflammatory drugs (NSAIDs) are often used in the management of chronic pain. Indeed, this group of drugs comprises the first step of the WHO analgesia ladder. Acetaminophen has minimal anti-inflammatory effect and lacks the side effect profile of the NSAIDs. Chronic high dosing can produce renal damage. Salicylates, such as aspirin, in high doses cause gastric irritation, which often limits their use clinically. Also, aspirin at any dose interferes with platelet function, which can lead to bleeding problems.

As a group, the NSAIDs produce similar adverse effects, but the frequency and severity vary with the individual and the specific drug. The major toxicities of the NSAIDs are gastrointestinal, hematologic, renal, and central nervous system (table 9.3).

All NSAIDs can cause dyspepsia and untoward gastrointestinal effects,

TABLE 9.3 The Clinically Important
Side Effects of Nonsteroidal
Anti-Inflammatory Drugs

Gastrointestinal irritation and ulceration
Bleeding due to platelet dysfunction
Impaired renal function
CNS toxicity, including dizziness, anxiety,
drowsiness, tinnitus, and confusion

Sources: Medical Letter (1989b); Enck (1991);
Wolfe, Lichenstein, and Singh (1999).

including bleeding, ulceration, and perforation in patients treated
chronically with these drugs (Wolfe, Lichenstein, and Singh 1999). They
interfere with platelet function and can cause bleeding. NSAIDs decrease
renal blood flow, cause fluid retention, and may cause renal failure in
some patients, especially elderly people. All NSAIDs can cause dizziness,
anxiety, drowsiness, tinnitus, and confusion, which may occur initially
and disappear with further use. Other less common side effects, such as
hepatitis, pancreatitis, and the like, have also been noted (*Medical Letter*
1989b).

Summary

To prevent the development of drug-induced side effects, physicians
must recognize and address factors such as age, impaired pulmonary
function, and the like during therapy for pain management. A minority
of patients treated by the WHO analgesia ladder experience no side effects. Strong opioids (namely, morphine) produce more side effects than
do either nonopioids or weak opioids. Finally, NSAIDs are frequently
used in managing pain, but their role is often limited by side effects, especially gastrointestinal distress.

Tolerance seems to develop in all patients receiving opioids on a
chronic basis and may occur after a week or more of morphine therapy.
It is important for the clinician to understand physical dependence because of the occurrence of withdrawal symptoms, which may be subtle or
significant, depending on the duration and dosage of opioids being used
when these drugs are stopped. Clinically, this problem can be avoided by
a gradual decrease in the daily dosages of opioids. The incidence of addiction in cancer patients taking opioids chronically is probably no
greater than 0.1 percent and is not a valid reason for physicians to un-
dertreat patients with severe pain.

Chapter 10

Bone Pain

Bone pain due to cancer metastasis is common. The most frequent primary sites leading to bone metastases are the breast, lung, and prostate. Autopsy studies have identified bone metastases in up to 85 percent of patients dying of these cancers. Most other primary tumor sites can spread to bone, including renal, thyroid, endometrial, cervical, bladder, and gastrointestinal tract cancers, but these sites account for less than 20 percent of patients with bone metastases. Although the presence of metastatic bone disease generally denotes a poor prognosis, a sizable proportion of these individuals will live for several months to years. For example, the median survival for patients with metastatic breast cancer is one to two years, but for subgroups of patients with bone metastasis only, a median survival of four years has been reported. The median survival of patients with metastatic prostate cancer is two years, but individual survival varies widely. In contrast, almost all patients with bone metastasis from lung cancer die within one year.

Pain, pathologic fractures, hypercalcemia, neurologic impairment, and immobility are the complications of bone metastases which adversely affect the quality of life for these patients. Neurologic deficits in the form of cranial nerve paralysis and headache are often seen in patients with tumor metastasis at the base of the skull. Involvement of the vertebral body and sacral bone may present diagnostic problems because metastases in these locations may cause not local but referred pain (Payne 1989b).

Pathophysiology

Tumor cells spread to bone mainly by the hematogenous route. In certain sites, direct invasion of bone may also occur. Oral or pharyngeal carcinomas may invade facial bones, and breast, lung, or esophageal tumors may directly involve the bony thorax. These tumors are usually ulcerating or pyogenic, since the bone periosteum is an effective barrier to closed noninfected cancers.

More than 80 percent of bone metastases are found in the axial skeleton because of the high distribution of red marrow in these bones. The spine, ribs, and pelvis are often the earliest site of metastases, whereas the skull, femora, humeri, scapulae, and sternum are involved later. Different primary tumors do not exhibit significant variation in their spread to bony sites, except that cancers of the prostate, bladder, cervix, and rectum tend to involve pelvic bones. Bone metastases are generally widespread by the time of their initial clinical presentation.

The destruction of bone is initially mediated by osteoclast-stimulating factors from the tumor or, more often, from the tumor-associated stroma or even the bone itself. In most carcinomas, the main factor is most likely a prostaglandin; in lymphoma and myeloma, it may be osteoclast-activating factor (OAF).

The relationship between bone invasion and bone pain is unclear. For example, 25 percent of patients with bone metastases have no symptoms; in the other 75 percent, however, pain is the main symptom. Postulated mechanisms that may cause pain from bone metastases include the following:

- stimulation of the nerve endings in the endosteum resulting from the destroyed bone's releasing a variety of chemical agents such as prostaglandin, bradykinin, substance P, or histamine;
- periosteal stretching by enlarging tumors;
- fracture; and
- extension of the tumor into the surrounding nerve and tissues.

Stimulation of endosteal nerve endings by released chemical agents is probably the dominant mechanism of bone pain from small metastases. As these metastases enlarge, stretching of the periosteum also contributes to the pain (Nielsen, Munro, and Tannock 1991).

Radiation Therapy

The management of a patient with painful bone metastases from advanced cancer generally involves more than one therapeutic approach to reach the goal of adequate pain control. When the clinician has identified painful sites of bone metastases, he or she should consider localized radiotherapy. With this modality, palliation is achieved for 70 to 100 percent of patients (Poulsen et al. 1989). The available data suggest that, for most patients, local radiotherapy for painful localized bone metastases can be given as a single treatment of 8 Gy (Poulsen et al. 1989; Nielsen, Munro, and Tannock 1991; McQuay 1998).

The biologic basis by which radiotherapy relieves bone pain is unknown. This is underscored by the observation that some patients experience relief of pain within 48 hours of a single dose, whereas other patients do not achieve relief until two to eight weeks after treatment.

Radioactive isotopes, which deliver radiation systemically, have been administered for widespread involvement of bone. The bone-seeking isotope strontium-89 in several studies showed overall frequencies of pain relief of approximately 58 percent. However, the time to response is longer; therefore strontium-89 is not appropriate for the dying patient (Editorial 1990b). Two additional agents used for bone pain palliation are rhenium-186 etidronate and samarium-153 ethylenediaminetetramethylene phosphonate, both of which have response rates comparable to that of strontium-89 (Chatal and Hoefnagel 1999). Pain relief obtained with radioactive isotopes is similar to that achieved with hemibody radiation without the added risk of gastrointestinal or pulmonary toxicity.

Pharmacotherapy

NONSTEROIDAL ANTI-INFLAMMATORY DRUGS

Nonsteroidal anti-inflammatory drugs (NSAIDs) are often used for analgesic therapy for painful bone metastases. The NSAIDs, theoretically, block the synthesis of prostaglandin, which, in turn, obviates the role of prostaglandin in the destruction of bone and the stimulation of endosteal nerve endings. A study by Levick et al. (1988) compared the safety and efficacy of two dosages of naproxen sodium in 100 patients with bone pain due to metastatic cancer. In approximately 80 percent of the patients, either 550 mg of naproxen sodium orally three times a day or 275 mg orally three times a day provided relief from pain. Subsequent treatment on the high-dose regimen was more effective than the low-dose regimen in reducing the pain of bone metastases. Both regimens were equally tolerated; however, gastrointestinal complaints were reported in 7 percent on the low dose and 16 percent on the high dose.

In a related study, Toscani et al. (1989) used a subcutaneous continuous infusion of naproxen sodium in 14 patients with advanced cancer; these patients were unable to tolerate oral medication. Ten of the 14 patients (71%) had bone pain. The mean duration of the continuous subcutaneous infusion was 21 days, with a range of 7 to 112 days. In four patients, naproxen was combined with continuous morphine infusion, with a mean daily dose of naproxen of 1,100 mg. Ten patients were given naproxen only at a mean daily dose of 1,375 mg. No pain or burning was noted at the infusion site, nor did intolerance or local or generalized reactions to naproxen occur. The same level of pain control achieved by prior oral naproxen administration was maintained for all patients.

Other NSAIDs, such as ketoprofen, indomethacin, and ibuprofen, may be effective in reducing pain due to metastatic bone disease (Payne 1989b; Phillips 1998).

BISPHOSPHONATES

Bisphosphonates provide another method of treating bone metastases systemically. These agents, such as amidronate (APD), inhibit osteoclasts. In a randomized trial, Van Holten-Verzantvoort et al. (1987) studied the use of oral APD in 131 women with bone metastases from breast cancer. An interim analysis revealed a significant reduction in pathologic fractures and severe bone pain in the APD-treated group. Gastrointestinal side effects of APD, mainly nausea, led 8 percent of the patients to drop out of the study. Subsequently, the medical literature shows that the clinical use of bisphosphonates, predominantly pamidronate, in patients with metastatic bone disease dramatically increased, as reflected in the medical literature. To provide guidelines for physicians, the American Society of Clinical Oncology assembled an expert panel to review pertinent information from the published literature and meeting abstracts through May 1999 (Hillner et al. 2000). The panel found that bisphosphonates have not had an impact on patient survival. The benefits have been reductions in skeletal complications (i.e., pathologic fracture), surgery for fracture or impending fracture, radiation, spinal cord compression, and hypercalcemia. The panel recommended that current standards of care for cancer pain, analgesics and localized radiation therapy, not be displaced by bisphosphonates. Intravenous pamidronate was associated with only a modest pain control benefit in controlled trials of women with metastatic bone disease due to breast cancer. Therefore, pamidronate should be used concurrently with systemic chemotherapy and/or hormonal therapy for these patients to relieve pain. The panel concluded that bisphosphonates provide a meaningful supportive but not life-prolonging benefit to many patients with bone metastases from cancer, and it encouraged further research on the use of these agents.

STEROIDS

Tannock et al. (1989) used low-dose prednisone (7.5 to 10 mg daily) to treat 37 males with prostatic cancer that had not been cured by prior therapy with estrogens and/or orchiectomy. The response to treatment was assessed by serial pain measurement instruments. Fourteen patients (38%) showed improvement in these scales used to measure pain at one month after starting prednisone, and 7 patients (19%) maintained this improvement for 3 to 30 months, with a median of 4 months. This reduction in pain was associated with an improvement in other dimensions of the quality of life as well as in overall well-being.

Summary

Bone metastases are common among patients with breast, lung, or prostate cancer and are often the source of severe, unrelenting pain. Local radiotherapy, given as a single treatment of 8 Gy, is effective palliation for painful localized bone metastases. The NSAIDs are the initial analgesic therapy to manage bone pain, but their usefulness is often limited by gastrointestinal toxicity. Low-dose prednisone may be useful in alleviating pain from metastatic bone disease for patients with prostatic cancer that has failed to respond to hormonal manipulation. Bisphosphonates, such as intravenous pamidronate, can prevent the skeletal complications of metastatic bone disease but should be used in combination with systemic cancer therapies to relieve pain.

Chapter 11

Surgery and Other Nonpharmacologic Interventions to Manage Pain

Surgery

Neurosurgical intervention provides an important alternative in the management of severe pain. The use of nerve blocks and neuroablative procedures to relieve pain has declined with the advent and refinement of the oral administration of opioids. Furthermore, neuroablation is not always permanent or always successful and has a high incidence of side effects (fig. 11.1). Indications for nerve blocks (Ferrer-Brechner 1989; Hanks and Justins 1992; Sykes, Johnson, and Hanks 1997) (table 11.1) are the following:

- pain responding to opioid analgesics, with an anticipated outcome of reducing doses and side effects and enhancing pain relief;
- pain not responding to opioid analgesics and control of psychological factors;
- specific pain (e.g., that from pancreatic carcinoma or pathologic rib fracture);
- the need for bodily functions important to the patient to be spared by the procedure; and
- a risk-to-benefit ratio acceptable to patients, families, and physicians.

Nondestructive nerve blocks involve the local injection of long-acting anesthetics, such as bupivacaine, or steroids and can be useful in determining the results of the destructive block intended. Local anesthetic can block central, epidural, peripheral (somatic and sympathetic), or visceral (celiac plexus) pain.

Destructive nerve blocks involve the injection of neurolytic solutions, such as alcohol and phenol, and the injection of freezing probes into nerves or ganglia. Neurolytic agents produce variable, nonselective nerve damage with a poor correlation between histologic damage and pain

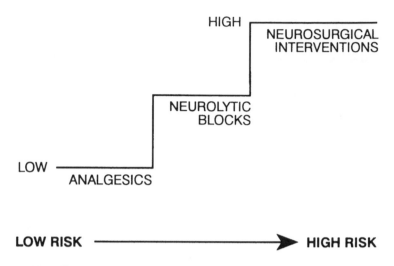

Figure 11.1. The risk related to neuroablative procedures

relief. The blocks are not permanent and last from hours to months (Ferrer-Brechner 1989). There is a high incidence of complications, including damage to adjacent structures, neuralgia, motor weakness, and autonomic dysfunction (such as incontinence), which, according to Hanks and Justins (1992) creates an unfavorable risk-to-benefit ratio. In a divergent opinion, from the viewpoint of a pain clinic, Wells (1989) suggested that neurolytic procedures are underused. He reported that, in his experience as director of the Center for Pain Relief in Liverpool, United Kingdom, 83 percent of patients referred with cancer pain experienced pain control with medication alone. Of the remaining 17 percent of patients, 13 percent were successfully treated by nerve block.

Sharp and Stevens (1991) reported their experience in using intraoperative celiac plexus block for pain relief for patients with cancer of the pancreas. All patients had operative celiac plexus block with absolute alcohol at the time of exploratory laparotomy for biliary bypass, gastroenterostomy, or biopsy of tumor. Ten of the 12 patients obtained complete postoperative pain relief, and only 2 had partial pain relief. There were no operative complications related to the celiac plexus block. The mean postoperative survival was 3.5 months, and most patients had excellent pain relief for at least 2 months or until death.

A short life expectancy does not limit the use of neurosurgical procedures (Wells 1989; Hanks and Justins 1992), but this approach is associated with significant neurologic complications and morbidity. Cordotomy is the most widely used and effective neuroablative procedure (Sundaresan, DiGiacinto, and Hughes 1989); the pain fibers in the an-

TABLE 11.1   The Indications for Nerve
Blocks to Control Pain

Reduction in doses and side effects, and en-
   hanced pain relief in opioid-responsive
   pain
Pain not responsive to opioid analgesics
Site-specific pain
   Pancreatic cancer
   Pathologic rib fracture
Preservation of important bodily functions
A risk-to-benefit ratio acceptable to patients,
   families, and physicians

Sources: Ferrer-Brechner (1989); Hanks and
Justins (1992); Sykes, Johnson, and Hanks
(1997).

terolateral quadrant of the spinal cord are interrupted, thus avoiding significant sensory and motor loss. Percutaneous cordotomy is the most frequent procedure and consists of creating a lesion in the anterolateral
spinal cord at the C1–2 level by inserting a needle with radiofrequency
current (fig. 11.2).

Sundaresan, DiGiacinto, and Hughes (1989) summarized the results
of the five largest series of unilateral percutaneous cordotomies performed in cancer patients. In the 648 patients, the initial success rate was
high, ranging from 71 to 98 percent, but after one to two years failures
were common, with declining analgesia and, often, dysesthesia. Morbidity ranged from 0 to 9 percent. Complications occurred, of which respiratory depression was the most serious, since the respiratory fibers are located deep in the anterolateral quadrant. As noted by Wells (1989), the
clinician must take care when continuing to give oral opioids after percutaneous anterolateral cordotomy, since these drugs may enhance the
problem of postoperative respiratory depression. In addition to respiratory difficulties (range of 0 to 6%), long-term bladder dysfunction (range
of 0 to 7%) and weakness (range of 0 to 10%) were other complications
of percutaneous cordotomy (Sundaresan, DiGiacinto, and Hughes 1989).

Indications for percutaneous cordotomy (Sundaresan, DiGiacinto,
and Hughes 1989; Wells 1989; Hanks and Justins 1992) (table 11.2) are:

- unilateral pain in patients when a reasonable attempt has been made
  to control the pain by the use of analgesic drugs,
- unilateral leg pain due to lumbosacral plexopathy caused by rectal
  or gynecologic cancer, and
- mesothelioma.

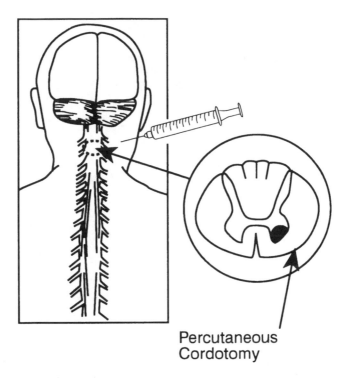

**Percutaneous
Cordotomy**

Figure 11.2. The procedure for percutaneous cordotomy

Other, less frequently used surgical neuroablative procedures include the creation of dorsal root entry zone lesion, midline commissural myelotomy, dorsal rhizotomy, hypophysectomy, medullary tractotomy, and stereotactic procedures (Sundaresan, DiGiacinto, and Hughes 1989).

Unlike neuroablation, neuroaugmentative procedures stimulate endogenous pain-modulating or pain-suppressing systems within the central nervous system. Electrodes and pulse generators can stimulate appropriate spinal cord, brainstem, and cortical structures. This procedure has been effective in selected patients with arachnoiditis and other neuropathic pain problems (Peters 1997). Although there is little experience with this technique in cancer-related pain, spinal stimulation has a potential role for patients with severe neuropathic pain from epidural or major nerve plexus involvement or radiation-induced neuritis. Complications include infection, migration or fracture of leads, and failure of the generator (Lamer 1994).

TABLE 11.2   The Indications for Percutaneous Cordotomy to Control Pain

Unilateral opioid-resistant pain
Unilateral lower extremity pain caused by lumbosacral plexus involvement by rectal and gynecologic cancers
Mesothelioma

Sources: Sundaresan, DiGiacinto, and Hughes (1989); Wells (1989); Hanks and Justins (1992).

Acupuncture

Acupuncture started in China during the Stone Age. Flint needles were used, and the evidence was recorded on tortoise shells. Huang Ti, or the Yellow Emperor, reigned in approximately 2600 B.C. Ti wanted to pass on the secrets of medicine to his sons and grandsons. To this end, *The Yellow Emperor's Classic of Internal Medicine* (Veith 1972) was written sometime between 475 and 221 B.C. The Yellow Emperor thought that the balance of Yin and Yang, forces of opposite polarities present in nature, was the basic principle of the entire universe. These forces—positive and negative, light and dark, masculine and feminine—should be present in appropriate amounts in each organ for healthy function.

The authors of *The Yellow Emperor's Classic* were strongly influenced by the beliefs of Lao-Tse, who had been born in 604 B.C. and from whom the religion of Taoism sprang. Taoism is based on scriptures from Lao-Tse called *Tao-te-ching* or *The Book of Change*. Lao espoused the concept of Yin and Yang dynamism and balance in all aspects of life. Sickness is viewed as no more than an artificial separation from the life-giving and abundant energizers of the universe. To achieve health, the individual must restore the harmony and connection of these universal energizers with currents of the same energizers (Powell 1979).

The Chinese described a circulation of vital energy, Qi, with deep and superficial components. When Qi gels, it causes life, but when dispersed it causes death. Qi travels throughout the body along meridians to nourish Yin and Yang of the various internal organs. These meridians are invisible lines joining a series of acupuncture points on the surface of the body.

The classification of acupuncture points has evolved over centuries. Any imbalance in the circulation of Qi could cause pain and disease. After taking a history and using a sophisticated pulse diagnosis, a physician could diagnose disease in 12 organs. The imbalance of energy could then be corrected by the insertion of needles into specifically chosen acupuncture points.

Despite centuries of use and decades of research, the precise mechanism of action of acupuncture in relieving pain remains unknown. As speculated by Filshie and Morrison (1988), acupuncture may work partly by involving natural pain-inhibitory pathways such as endogenous opioids and by nonopioid neurohumeral mechanisms.

Few studies have been done on the use of acupuncture in the management of chronic pain for terminally ill patients. In the largest series, Filshie and Redman (1985) treated 183 cancer patients with acupuncture and found that more than half (52%) of the patients whose pain had not responded to conventional treatment were helped. The initial pain relief response to acupuncture was high (82%), but the relief was short-lived, from several hours to several days, in 30 percent of the responding patients. All patients required multiple treatments, often one to four times weekly. The investigators found acupuncture especially effective for pain due to vascular problems, dysesthetic conditions, muscle spasm, and metastatic bone disease.

Transcutaneous Electrical Nerve Stimulation

Transcutaneous electrical nerve stimulation (TENS) has been used for acute and chronic pain in a wide variety of settings, with varied results. TENS employs an electrical current applied to the skin to reduce or abolish the sensation of pain. Similar to acupuncture, TENS may stimulate the release of endogenous pain-relieving opioids. Unlike acupuncture, however, TENS may have longer-lasting effects.

In 1988, Librach and Rapson reviewed the medical literature over a 15-year period on the use of TENS in the treatment of cancer pain. They found scant research specifically investigating the use of TENS in cancer pain and found no investigative papers of this type in the literature on palliative care. One of the few descriptive studies (Avellanosa and West 1982) reported on 60 patients with cancer pain. After two weeks of treatment with TENS, there was an excellent response in 28 percent of patients, a fair response in 37 percent, and a failure to respond in 35 percent. After three months, however, these response rates were 15 percent, 18 percent, and 67 percent, respectively, showing a decline in response to placebo levels. The response of patients with bodily and extremity pain, especially arm pain, was better than the response of patients with pelvic or visceral pain. Overall, Librach and Rapson (1988) thought that the evidence documenting the effectiveness of TENS in cancer pain was spare and inconclusive. Furthermore, Jacox et al. (1994) suggested that part of the efficacy of TENS is related to a placebo effect, but patients with mild pain may benefit from a trial of TENS therapy.

Relaxation Techniques

The use of relaxation techniques in the acute pain setting is well appreciated (Acute Pain Management Guideline Panel 1992), but information is lacking on its use and efficacy in the dying patient with chronic pain. Some of the inherent difficulties in engaging these relaxation techniques in terminally ill patients are the cognitive function of the patient, length of time necessary to learn these approaches, and need for skilled personnel to teach them.

Complementary/Alternative Medicine

In 1998, Ernst and Cassileth studied the prevalence rate of the use of complementary/alternative medicine (CAM) in the treatment of cancer. A series of computerized literature searches identified 26 surveys from 13 countries, including 4 studies of pediatric patients. The use of CAM therapies in adult populations ranged from 7 to 64 percent. The mean prevalence across all adult patients was 31.4 percent. These treatments varied from laetrile in the 1970s to the recently popular holistic therapies. In a survey of 453 patients at the University of Texas M.D. Anderson Cancer Center, Richardson et al. (2000) found that the use of multiple CAM therapies with conventional treatment was widespread, disclosure to physicians was low, and the desire for information about CAM was high. Among the patients who had heard of CAM, the use of at least one CAM modality was 83 percent. The most popular CAM therapies were spiritual practices, vitamins and herbs, movement and physical therapies, and mind/body approaches. Richardson et al. (2000) confirmed that the stereotype of the terminally ill, desperate, uneducated patient using CAM was inaccurate. Furthermore, patients with advanced disease were more likely to use CAM because their disease was incurable and were less likely to expect symptom relief from these alternative therapies.

Despite the widespread use of CAM, there have been no scientific studies on the effectiveness of this modality in the treatment of pain or other symptoms in the dying patient. Herbs such as external capsicum, sunflower seeds, willow bark tea, and mountain leaf tea are often used (Cassileth 1999) but again, scientific support is lacking.

Summary

Nerve blocks and neuroablative procedures are important options in the management of pain. Nerve blocks are generally used for opioid-responsive pain when side effects are unmanageable and intolerable or for severe pain that does not respond to opioids. The use of an intraoperative celiac plexus block to relieve pain in patients with cancer of the pancreas is a good example of site-specific pain ablation. Radical neurosurgical procedures such as percutaneous cordotomy are rarely done, which attests to the effectiveness of oral opioids in controlling pain.

For other nonpharmacologic interventions—namely, acupuncture, transcutaneous electrical nerve stimulation, relaxation techniques, and complementary/alternative medicine—scant scientific information exists to support their widespread use in the management of chronic pain for the dying patient.

PART III

The Management of Symptoms during the Last Few Days

Chapter 12

The Final Moments

Death due to chronic illness, such as cancer, is rarely rapid. Dying usually lasts a few hours to days. It is a continuous process as the body and brain are unable to cope with hypoxia, malnutrition, electrolyte imbalance, tumor burden, and toxins that are not cleared from the body as hepatic and renal failure occur. Emotion, cognition, thinking, behavior, and autonomic function all slowly deteriorate, and, in most cases, coma ensues before death.

Two roads to coma have been described in the dying patient: the high road and the low road. The low road is the more common and is a path of increasing sedation to coma and death. This path does not seem to be traumatic for patients, and surviving friends and relatives generally recall a peaceful death. If not controlled, the high road is much more traumatic, resembling the organic brain syndrome of delirium. Symptoms of this organic brain syndrome include restlessness, confusion, agitation, hallucinations, myoclonic jerks, seizures, and finally coma. A preterminal delirium can start as many as nine days before death. Over time, the symptoms often become increasingly severe, and surviving family members frequently remember a terrible death even when the symptoms were well controlled up until the preterminal delirium (Ferris 1990).

Terminal Symptoms and Their Management

Lichter and Hunt (1990) designed a study to document the problems that arose during the last days in the life of terminally ill cancer patients and to record their frequency and the management used. Based on a pilot study, they chose a time frame of 48 hours because it was during this period that symptoms most commonly occurred in patients who had previously been comfortable.

Two hundred consecutive patients at the Te Omanga Hospice, in Lower Hutt, New Zealand, were studied. A patient record was established and maintained by the nurses when it was thought that the patient was likely to die or whenever terminal symptoms such as twitching, jerking, restlessness, agitation, and plucking were observed. The presence of other symptoms was also recorded, and observations were continued until the patient's death. In some cases, this was longer than 48 hours, and in these instances only the features occurring in the last 48 hours were analyzed.

The results of the study showed that 36 percent of patients experienced some problems in the last 48 hours of life. The great majority of patients (91.5%) died peacefully. Factors that interfered with a peaceful death in a few patients (8.5%) were hemorrhage and hemoptysis, respiratory distress, restlessness, pain, myocardial infarction, and regurgitation.

Slightly more than half (51%) of the patients experienced pain in the last 48 hours (table 12.1). Strict pain criteria were used, and every headache, backache, pressure area pain, movement pain, or transient discomfort noted at any time during the last 48 hours was recorded as pain. New pain was noted in 29.5 percent of the patients, and exacerbation of previously controlled pain occurred in 21.5 percent of patients.

Of all the patients, 91 percent were taking opioid analgesics and 25 percent were taking nonsteroidal anti-inflammatory drugs. Approximately the same number of patients required no change (39%) or an increased opioid dosage (40%) during the last 48 hours. In only 12 percent was the dosage of opioids decreased. Pain was not completely controlled in 10 percent of the patients, but no patient experienced persistent, severe pain.

Movement-related or disturbance pain was identified in 18 percent of the patients. This discomfort was noted even in comatose patients, who would moan or cry out when moved. It was suggested that this pain was related to joint stiffness and muscle weakness and that it can be eased by gentle passive movement at an earlier stage. Also, analgesics can be given before any major disturbance such as sponging.

Dyspnea occurred in 22 percent of the patients. The goal of treating terminal dyspnea is to relieve the perception of breathlessness. Dyspnea causing distress is generally associated with tachypnea accompanied by anxiety. A draft of cool air is helpful in alleviating this shortness of breath and can be achieved by opening a window or using a fan. It is thought that the perception of breathlessness is altered by stimulating receptors in the distribution of the trigeminal nerve in the cheek. Also, the passage of cool air into the nasal cavity relieves dyspnea by further stimulating other trigeminal nerve receptors in the nasopharynx. If additional measures are needed, a benzodiazepine can be administered. The perception of breathlessness can also be relieved by reducing the rate of breathing to a comfortable level using morphine. The dosage of morphine is

Table 12.1 The Frequency of Symptoms and Their Management during the Last 48 Hours of Life

Symptom	Frequency (%)	Management
Noisy and moist breathing	56	Atropine or scopolamine (0.4 mg repeated every 4–8h as needed) along with morphine (10–15 mg)
		Suctioning, change of position, and reassurance
Pain	51	Adjustment in opioid dosage
Restlessness and agitation	42	Methotrimeprazine (25–50 mg IM every 4h as needed)
		Diazepam (5–10 mg)
		Chlorpromazine (50 mg every 4–8 hours)
		Midazolam (10 mg stat dose and then starting dose of 30 mg/day using continuous infusion)
		Lorazepam (sublingually in doses of 1–2 mg every hour as needed)
Urinary incontinence	32 and	Padding
retention	21	Male external catheter
		Indwelling catheter
Difficulty swallowing	29	Rectal administration of drugs
		Continuous infusion of medications, preferably subcutaneous, via pump device
Dyspnea	22	Reassurance
		Bedside fan
		Diazepam (5–10 mg stat dose and then 5–20 mg at night)
		Morphine (5–10 mg every 4h or doses of morphine titrated to achieve a respiratory rate of 15–20 respirations/min)
Nausea and vomiting	14	Antiemetics, such as haloperidol, administered by continuous infusion
Sweating and feeling of heat	14	Steroids
		Indomethacin (100 mg rectally)
Muscle twitching, jerking and		Diazepam
plucking	12	Midazolam (5 mg stat dose and starting dose of 10 mg/day by continuous infusion as muscle relaxant; 5 mg stat dose and starting dose of 20 mg/day by continuous infusion for multifocal myoclonus)
Confusion	9	Reassurance
		Haloperidol (5–10 mg IM stat dose, then oral or IM 5–15 mg daily)
		Chlorpromazine (50 mg)

Sources: Data from Saunders (1982); Lichter and Hunt (1990); Adam (1997).

titrated against the respiratory rate to obtain a rate of 15 to 20 respirations per minute. Patients already receiving morphine for pain usually require an approximately 50 percent increase in dosage to achieve a suitable reduction in respiratory rate. Of the 22 percent of patients experiencing terminal dyspnea, all but 2 percent responded to treatment with morphine and a benzodiazepine, usually very promptly.

Noisy and moist breathing was present in 56 percent of the patients. Although not distressful to the patient, moist respiration or the death rattle was troubling to relatives and caregivers. Anticholinergic drugs such as atropine or scopolamine (0.4 mg) were effective if existing secretions in the back of the throat were first cleared. Noisy respiration requiring medication was noted in 25 percent of patients. Anticholinergic drugs were immediately successful in 94 percent of these patients, and 6 percent required repeated doses. A further 31 percent needed only nursing interventions, which included suctioning, change of position, and reassurance.

Nausea and vomiting were noted in only 14 percent of the patients. In 6 percent it was a continuation or exacerbation of previously existing nausea and vomiting, and in 8 percent it was a new symptom. For exacerbations, increases in continuously infused antiemetics were needed. In some patients, treatment of constipation relieved this symptom.

Nine percent of the patients experienced confusion in the last 48 hours. Confusion was best managed by reassurance. Restraints were not used; instead, constant supervision was maintained. When the confusion was marked, drug treatment was added. Haloperidol (5 to 10 mg intramuscular immediately and then oral administration, or intramuscular 5 to 15 mg daily) was helpful, especially in the presence of hallucinations or paranoia. Benzodiazepines were useful when the patient was restless and agitated, although they may have a paradoxical effect and increase restlessness. Chlorpromazine (dose of 50 to 100 mg) was sometimes successful when haloperidol failed and was particularly useful when sedation was needed.

Restlessness and agitation occurred frequently (42%). For relieving restlessness, methotrimeprazine (25 to 50 mg given intramuscularly and repeated every four hours as needed), which has both analgesic and antiemetic properties, was used. If the restlessness was not controlled, the addition of a benzodiazepine such as diazepam was often effective. An alternative was chlorpromazine. These drugs singly or in combination relieved restlessness in all patients. In 5 percent of patients, a change of medication was successful when the drug of first choice was not effective.

Muscle twitching and jerking was identified in 12 percent of the patients. The treatment of choice was benzodiazepines and anticonvulsants, and all patients obtained good relief.

Urinary incontinence and the retention of urine were recorded in 32 percent and 21 percent of the patients, respectively. An indwelling catheter was used in 44 percent, and a male external catheter was used in 4 percent. A common cause of difficulty of micturition was the presence of rectal feces, which was managed by suppository, enema, or manual removal.

Sweating occurred in 14 percent of the patients and was usually managed with steroids and indomethacin.

Finally, the authors studied the time duration of consciousness. Thirty percent of the patients were conscious until death, 38 percent became unconscious from 0 to 12 hours before death, 24 percent became unconscious from 12 to 24 hours before death, 7 percent became unconscious 24 to 48 hours before death, and 1 percent were unconscious for more than 48 hours.

To determine the physical and medical changes in the dying process, Morita et al. (1998) conducted a prospective study on 100 terminally ill cancer patients admitted to the Seirei Hospice in Japan. Fifty-five of the patients were men and 45 of the patients were women, with a mean age of 67 years. The mean length of stay at the hospice was 43 days. More than half (63%) of the patients had cancer of either the gastrointestinal tract or the lung. Clinical signs that suggested impending death included clouding of the consciousness, death rattle, respiration with mandibular movement (RMM), cyanotic extremities, and pulselessness on the radial artery. Opioid consumption and additional use of opioid or nonopioid medications were recorded daily. RMM, cyanosis of the extremities, and death rattle were observed before death in 95 percent, 80 percent, and 35 percent of the patients, respectively. The mean times from onset of death rattle, RMM, cyanosis, and pulselessness on the radial artery to death were 57 hours, 7.6 hours, 5.1 hours, and 2.6 hours, respectively. Death rattle was observed significantly earlier than were the other signs, and RMM was noted earlier than pulselessness. Thus, in many patients, as death approached, death rattle was observed first, RMM began second, and cyanosis of the extremities and pulselessness of the radial artery followed, resulting in death within a few hours. However, the intervals from each episode until the time of death varied widely among the patients. Fifty percent of the patients were unconscious in the final 6 hours, whereas 12 percent were unconscious in the last 24 hours, and none was unconscious one week before death. The mean dose of opioids increased significantly as death approached, from 49 mg/day (parenteral morphine equivalents) 4 weeks before death to 139 mg/day in the final 48 hours. The frequency of additional doses also increased significantly, from 32 percent (opioid) and 40 percent (nonopioid) one week before death to 68 percent and 66 percent in the last 48 hours. Based on their study, the authors concluded that changing physical signs when death is impending have a common pathway; however, it is difficult to predict precisely the time of death according to these signs because of large individual variation. Furthermore, nearly two-thirds of patients required additional pain medication during the final 48 hours.

Due to the need for escalating doses of opioids as death nears and the concern that this may shorten patients' lives, Thorns and Sykes (2000) retrospectively studied 238 consecutive patients admitted to a 62-bed hospice unit. The median inpatient stay was 9 days and the mean age of the patients was 69 years. The authors reported that patients who received opioid increases at the end of life did not show a shorter survival than those who received no increases. Furthermore, the doctrine of double effect—defined as a harmful effect of treatment, even resulting in death, which is permissible if it is not intended and occurs as a side effect of a beneficial action—is not applicable in providing symptom control at the end of life.

Sublingual Lorazepam

To prevent hospitalization and maintain the patient at home, sublingual lorazepam and continuous subcutaneous infusions of midazolam have been used to control restlessness and other terminal symptoms. Ferris (1990) suggested the use of sublingual lorazepam as an alternative to haloperidol for dying patients unable to swallow. This route also obviates the need for intermittent painful injections and is well suited for the home care setting. Lorazepam is given sublingually in doses of 1 to 2 mg every hour as needed with a few drops of water, and the dosage is increased to 2 to 4 mg every hour as needed. Sedation occurs in most patients after a few milligrams, and subsequent doses can be administered when symptoms recur.

Midazolam

Amesbury and Dunphy (1989) used continuous subcutaneous infusions of midazolam to manage terminal restlessness in six patients cared for at home. Midazolam is a short-acting, water-soluble benzodiazepine used as the sole induction agent, in some cases, for anesthesia and frequently used for sedation, especially when amnesia is desirable. All six patients had advanced cancer. Their mean age was 65 years, with a range of 45 to 84 years. A continuous infusion pump was used because the patients were experiencing episodes of reduced consciousness that made it difficult to swallow medication for pain and/or nausea and vomiting. In all cases, the infusion was continued until death, with a mean duration of 64 hours and a range of 24 to 216 hours. The mean total daily dose of midazolam was 30 mg, with a range of 20 to 40 mg. When the midazolam infusion was added, the restlessness ceased in all cases. No side effects were noted with its use in this setting.

In a related paper, McNamara, Minton, and Twycross (1991) retrospectively studied the use of midazolam in 104 terminally ill patients. In 3 patients midazolam was administered intravenously as sedation for minor procedures; in 1 patient it was used intermittently subcutaneously as short-term sedation pending epidural analgesia. The 100 remaining patients received midazolam by continuous subcutaneous infusion for terminal agitation (61), muscle stiffness (27), multifocal myoclonus (7), and seizure prophylaxis (5). The median age of these 100 patients was 69 years, with a range of 26 to 89 years. The median dose was 30 mg/24 hours, and only 6 of 61 patients with terminal agitation required more than 100 mg/24 hours. No clinically relevant episodes of respiratory depression occurred, despite the fact that midazolam was often given in conjunction with opioids. No skin irritation was noted, even at the highest dose used, 240 mg/24 hours.

In the investigators' experience, midazolam was a safe and effective drug in the terminal setting. Based on this, they offered the following guidelines for the use of midazolam:

- as a muscle relaxant (5 mg stat dose, starting infusion rate of 10 mg/ 24 hours, common range of 10 to 30 mg/24 hours);
- for terminal agitation (10 mg stat dose, starting infusion rate of 30 mg/24 hours, common range of 30 to 60 mg/24 hours);
- as an anticonvulsant, including multifocal myoclonus (5 mg stat dose, starting infusion rate of 20 mg/24 hours, common range of 20 to 40 mg).

Berger et al. (2000) combined midazolam with ketamine and fentanyl to control pain and agitation successfully in 9 terminally ill patients with cancer. Ketamine (2 mg/ml), fentanyl (5 µg/ml), and midazolam (0.1 mg/ml) was continuously infused intravenously because increasing the dosage of opioids was ineffective in managing the patients' terminal symptoms. As reported by the authors, the patients died virtually pain free with little agitation.

Drug-Induced Terminal Sedation

As part of the National Hospice Study, Morris et al. (1986) studied the quality of life of terminally ill cancer patients. They collected data from two samples of cancer patients for the last 13 weeks of their lives. One sample consisted of patients followed in two hospital-based palliative care units in Montreal as part of a controlled study by the McGill Cancer Center. The other sample comprised patients in six hospices in the United States participating in the National Hospice Study project funded by the Health Care Financing Administration.

Using this information, the investigators tested a series of hypotheses concerning the quality of life during the final 13 weeks. They proposed two general clinical scenarios. In the first, they postulated that the patient experienced a significant loss of quality of life over some weeks, which resulted in the unrelenting picture of functional decline and symptomatic distress. In the second, a loss of quality of life was depicted as sudden in onset and lasting the final one to two weeks. A wide array of measures of the quality of life were used in the study.

Not surprisingly, the data supported the second scenario: declines in the quality of life varied as a function of the patient's proximity to death, with rapid decline being limited to the last one to three weeks of life. Many patients were in extreme pain some nine weeks before death, whereas many others had little or no pain. As death approached, the distribution of patients in pain changed little, and there was no rapid rise in either the average levels of pain or the number of patients with extreme pain in the last one to three weeks of life. Finally, some 20 percent of the patients did not fall into the categories of having a very low quality of life, even in the week before death.

The finding of no dramatic change in pain as death approached, reported by Morris et al. (1986), was also reported by Higginson and McCarthy (1989). These latter investigators studied the symptoms of 86 patients referred to a district terminal care support team. Pain was the most common severe symptom, occurring in a little less than half of the referred patients. Pain control was improved after one week of care by the support team, and further improvement was maintained until death, with no patient dying in severe pain.

One possible conclusion from these studies is that the vast majority of terminally ill cancer patients are dying pain free after a short downhill clinical course that lasts only a few weeks. However, if this is valid, why the appearance in the medical literature of three articles (Ventafridda et al. 1990b; Fainsinger et al. 1991; Greene and Davis 1991) on the topic of terminal sedation for uncontrolled symptoms? One answer may be that the results of scientific inquiry do not always reflect the realities of terminal care. Another answer may be confusion regarding terminology such as *pain* and *suffering*, the definition of symptoms, and the like.

Ventafridda et al. (1990b) studied 120 terminally ill cancer patients prospectively entering a home care program organized by the Palliative

Care Division of the National Cancer Institute of Milan. The home care team consisted of five physicians, seven registered nurses, one psychologist, one social worker, and approximately 100 volunteers. All patients were treated for pain based on the World Health Organization guidelines. The intensity of symptoms was assessed by an endurable/unendurable scale as reported by the patient. When symptoms could not be relieved through specific or symptomatic treatment, the dosages of opioids (morphine, methadone) and/or strong tranquilizers (diazepam, chlorpromazine, haloperidol) were gradually increased until the symptoms were controlled. Before entry into the study, the patients and families were informed that it is always possible to control symptoms but that sometimes this can be accomplished only by reducing the patients' level of consciousness. Both patients and families expressed their consent to this therapeutic approach.

Of the 120 patients, 73 were men and 47 were women, with a median age of 65.5 years. Lung cancer was the most common diagnosis. During the entire period of home care, there were 123 episodes of symptoms characterized by the patients as unendurable. In slightly more than one-third of the patients, the symptoms were controlled through therapeutic intervention by the home care physician. These controllable symptoms included pain (60%) and dyspnea (40%). However, symptoms were not controlled in 52 percent of the patients despite active symptomatic treatment. These symptoms appeared on average two days before death. Symptom control in these patients was possible only by increasing the dosages of drugs, predominantly opioids and tranquilizers, until sedation or sleep occurred. This lowered level of consciousness was maintained until death and was carried out with the advance permission of the patient or on an ad hoc basis.

Of the 63 patients who required sedation for uncontrollable symptoms, 75 percent had only one symptom, 24 percent had two, and 1 percent had three. The majority of patients had either dyspnea (41%) or pain (39%), with fewer patients experiencing delirium (14%) or vomiting (6%). Dyspnea was most frequent in patients with lung and head and neck cancers, whereas pain occurred in patients with breast, gastrointestinal tract, colorectal, and male genitourinary tract cancers. Vomiting was seen in patients with cancer of the female genitourinary tract.

The etiology of these uncontrolled symptoms was also investigated. In slightly more than half of the cases with dyspnea, massive tumor invasion of the lung parenchyma was found. Pain was related to bone involvement in one-third of the cases, and delirium was frequently related to the presence of brain metastases. Finally, vomiting generally was correlated with the occurrence of inoperable gastrointestinal tract obstruction.

From the start of home care, the median length of survival was 25 days for patients in whom sedation was necessary and 23 days for the other patients. This difference was not statistically significant.

The investigators involved in this study thought that their results highlighted important information that has been neglected in the published literature, that is, more than 50 percent of terminally ill cancer patients will die with physical suffering that can be controlled only by sedation. Furthermore, the authors speculated that the onset of unendurable and uncontrollable symptoms was a good prognosticator of imminent death. Finally, the authors did address, to some degree, the ethical question of this approach and thought that it was correct only if the patient's wishes were respected.

In a related article, Greene and Davis (1991) reported their experience with 17 terminally ill patients for whom they used continuous intravenous barbiturates to control symptoms. The authors did a retrospective review of patients with terminal cancer in their community-based urology practice. During the years 1975 to 1989, 17 patients with terminal cancer who were very close to death were identified. All attempts at curative treatment had been exhausted, and standard methods of palliative therapy were insufficient. The 17 patients ranged in age from 56 to 86 years, with a mean of 69 years. The tumor sites included prostate (8), bladder (5), kidney (2), colon (1), and pancreas (1). Symptoms included pain in bone and soft tissue, prolonged vomiting, abdominal distension, seizures, fecal emesis, retention of urine, and restlessness. Fifteen of these 17 patients were experiencing some degree of pain.

Prerequisites for intravenous barbiturate therapy included the following:

- the patient had terminal cancer;
- all other palliative treatments were exhausted;
- death was imminent, that is, likely to occur within hours or days;
- a do-not-resuscitate order was in effect;
- the patient and all family members were in agreement;
- a family member was in attendance at the bedside at all times.

In the first nine patients, amobarbital sodium, a short-to intermediate-acting barbiturate, was used. Initial doses ranged from 20 to 215 mg/hour, depending on the patient's weight and overall condition. An average dose of 218 mg/hour was employed. Thiopental sodium, an ultra-short-acting barbiturate, was administered to the last eight patients and was preferred because of its short half-life and the ease with which the dosage could be controlled. The mean dose of thiopental required was 107 mg/hour.

Unfortunately, the investigators did not use any objective parameters to measure the patient's level of consciousness other than simple clinical observation. Four patients died without total somnolence, but somnolence developed over 6 to 24 hours in the remaining 13 patients. This reduced level of consciousness lasted from 2 hours to four days, averaging 23 hours. According to the investigators, the patients all died peacefully in their sleep.

The use of a single-agent barbiturate allowed the investigators to induce somnolence or pharmacologic hypnosis to dissociate the patient's consciousness from severe symptoms. To the investigators, it seemed logical to achieve a somnolent effect with the use of a hypnotic agent rather than to increase an opioid toward its limit of toxicity to produce sedation. Continuous intravenous barbiturate is accepted therapy in other areas of medical practice, such as in the control of intubated patients receiving ventilatory support. As in Ventafridda et al.'s (1990b) study, sedation therapy was done with the consent of the patients and families.

Addressing the issue of the appropriateness of physician-assisted suicide for terminally ill patients, Greene and Davis (1991) observed that when symptoms are successfully controlled, cancer patients find no need to ask for euthanasia as a means of escape. Furthermore, the investigators thought that any shortening of life was incident to their objective of relieving suffering in situations in which the extension of life had no meaning.

In response to the study by Ventafridda et al. (1990b), Fainsinger et al. (1991) reported their experience with terminal sedation to control symptoms at the Edmonton (Alberta) General Hospital. These investigators retrospectively reviewed 100 consecutive patients admitted for six days or more to a 14-bed palliative care unit. Of the 100 patients, 51 were men and 49 were women, with a mean age of 62 years. Carcinoma of the gastrointestinal tract was the most common diagnosis, and the mean duration of admission was 40 days. A review of patient charts was done to collect information on major symptoms requiring treatment, symptom control at admission and during each of the last seven days of life, drugs used, and changes that may have contributed to sedation. Of the 100 patients, 99 needed treatment for pain, 71 for nausea, 46 for dyspnea, and 39 for delirium. Visual analog scores were recorded twice daily for all patients to assess pain and symptoms. The evaluation of patient records and changes in medication (with particular reference to sedating drugs, increasing doses, and changes in level of consciousness) revealed that 6 of 99 patients (6%) with pain and 10 of 39 patients (26%) with delirium requiring increased treatment, likely resulting in their sedation to an unresponsive state during the last days of life. Thus, the authors concluded, only 16 of 100 patients (16%) required treatment for pain and delirium that would have caused sedation to achieve control of symptoms.

Although the characteristics of the patients in these two studies (Ventafridda et al. 1990b; Fainsinger et al. 1991) are similar, the results are strikingly different; that is, 52 percent versus 16 percent of terminally ill patients required sedation to control symptoms. Also, the studies used differing methodologies: Ventafridda et al. (1990b) prospectively studied their patients, whereas Fainsinger et al. (1991) opted for a retrospective review of the patients' charts. The inherent weakness of this retrospective approach may well explain the disparity of the findings of these two investigations.

As noted by Roy (1991) in an editorial commenting on Ventafridda et al.'s study, this question of sedation-induced unconsciousness raises many issues, including ethical ones. Roy (1990) argued that the agitated and restless patient does little to prepare himself or herself and the family for death. In this instance, death in a sleep and forgetting state can bring comfort and peace. On the other hand, the use of drugs as a blunderbuss at the end of life would be to write off patients at the very moment when they need the most sensitive and competent care.

Cherny (2000) reviewed the literature in the years after the initial publications on terminal sedation by Ventafridda et al. (1990b), Greene and Davis (1991), and Fainsinger et al. (1991). He identified several additional reports and found that the proportion of patients sedated for refractory symptoms varied from 26 to 43 percent and that 0 to 8 percent were sedated for pain. In addition, he urged all physicians to be more skilled in the management of patients with refractory terminal symptoms.

Morita et al. (2000) addressed the use of sedating therapy for patients with intractable psychological distress, an area not well studied. They found that only 1 of 248 patients (0.4%) received sedation for psychological suffering, whereas physical symptoms were relieved. More commonly, this approach was used to control physical discomfort such as dyspnea, agitated delirium, and pain. In this retrospective study from the Seirei Hospice in Japan, 20 of 248 (8%) consecutive hospice inpatients expressed the meaninglessness of their lives and requested treatment with sedation. There were 8 men and 12 women, with an average age of 58 years. All the patients had cancer, and they died a median of 1.5 days after sedation was started. The authors concluded that terminal sedation for psychological distress is extremely rare in their hospice, and they encouraged further research in this area.

Quill and Byock (2000) reviewed the overall concept of terminal sedation, defined as the use of high dosages of sedatives to relieve extremes of physical distress. The purpose of the medication is to render the patient unconscious in order to alleviate suffering and not to intentionally end life. Terminal sedation differs from the coma that commonly occurs as death is imminent and is also distinct from the sedating effects of high-dose opioid treatment to relieve severe pain. In contrast, terminal sedation involves an explicit decision to render the patient unconscious to control unbearable physical distress. This approach is often used in critical care practice to treat symptoms of suffocation in dying patients who are discontinuing mechanical ventilation.

Although legal precedents guiding terminal sedation are less clear than those involving other end-of-life decisions, the 1997 U.S. Supreme Court decision on assisted suicide suggested that this practice is permitted under current law. In addition, Justices O'Connor and Souter supported the use of medication to alleviate the pain and suffering of terminally ill patients, even to the point of causing unconsciousness or hastening death. Opponents of physician-assisted suicide cite terminal sedation as a preferable alternative because the physician does not directly or intentionally cause death.

In reviewing published guidelines for terminal sedation, Quill and Byock (2000) emphasized two important criteria for its use. The first is informed consent, which includes evaluating the patient's capacity to understand the treatment and the available alternatives. The presence or absence of underlying depression should be recognized because, if present, depression may cloud the patient's decision-making process. The second criterion is severe suffering by the patient that cannot be relieved by any other means. The main indication for terminal sedation is uncontrolled physical distress, such as dyspnea, delirium, seizures, or intractable pain. Based on the experience of Morita et al. (2000), psychological distress should be added to this list. Terminal sedation should be used only in most difficult cases and should include discussion and understanding of the complex clinical and ethical issues by the patient, family, physician, and clinical team.

Appropriate drugs for sedating include the following:

- midazolam (rapid, short-acting benzodiazepine),
- lorazepam (benzodiazepine),
- propofol (general anesthetic with ultrarapid onset and elimination),
- thiopental (ultrashort-acting barbiturate),
- pentobarbital (long-acting barbiturate), and
- phenobarbital (long-acting barbiturate).

One of these drugs is rapidly infused to achieve sedation and provide the patient comfort. The interval from initiation of the infusion to death is usually hours to days. When a dying patient requires sedation, the physician should continue opioids and other drugs to control symptoms in order to avoid the possibility of unobservable pain or opioid withdrawal. Opioids are not usually effective at inducing sedation and are not the medications of choice.

The controversy surrounding terminal sedation has subsided over the last decade, as its role in caring for the dying is better understood. Nonetheless, the advice Dame Cicely Saunders (1984) gave years ago is worth remembering: "A blanket ordering of what may be an overdose for a particular patient would hardly seem to be the way to end a long-term commitment to a patient's care on the part of his doctors and nurses. Drugs are used as fine instruments, and to turn to their use as a blunderbuss at the end would intimate a final attitude tantamount to 'writing off' the patient."

Summary

In the dying patient, death is preceded by either progressive sedation or the development of the organic brain syndrome, delirium. More than one-third of dying patients experience some difficulty during their last 48 hours of life, with noisy and moist breathing, pain, and agitation and restlessness being the most common. The great majority of these symptoms can be managed by reassurance or drug intervention. Sublingual lorazepam and the continuous subcutaneous infusion of midazolam are effective in controlling terminal restlessness.

A disparity exists in the medical literature regarding the extent of control of a patient's symptoms just before death. According to Ventafridda et al. (1990b), more than half of the patients they studied required drug-induced sedation to control symptoms, whereas Fainsinger et al. (1991) found that only 16 percent of their patients needed terminal sedation. Subsequent studies reported variation in patients sedated for refractory symptoms (26 to 43%) and uncontrolled pain (0 to 8%). The controversy surrounding terminal sedation has subsided over the last decade as its role in managing the dying patient is better understood.

Chapter 13

Issues concerning the Sustaining of Life

Do Not Resuscitate

In the past several years, intense interest has focused on the complexities of the decision not to resuscitate. The prerogative not to resuscitate is the patient's, and this instruction means that if cardiac and/or pulmonary arrest occurs, no therapeutic attempt is made to reverse these events, and death ensues. In 1983, the President's Commission for the Study of Ethical Problems in Medicine and Biomedical and Behavioral Research raised three critical points: (1) resuscitation is a very painful and intrusive procedure; (2) efforts to resuscitate a dying patient are successful in only approximately one attempt in three and, of those patients who survive initial efforts at resuscitation, only one-third are eventually discharged (those who are able to return home are often significantly impaired); and (3) the success of resuscitation efforts is generally difficult to assess without carrying out the full range of procedures. These facts suggest that physicians who carry out less aggressive efforts because they did not thoroughly consider the resuscitation decision ahead of time may not be acting in their patients' best interests.

Based on their deliberations, the President's Commission made three chief recommendations for the development of policies on resuscitation: (1) hospitals should develop explicit policies on the practice of writing and implementing do-not-resuscitate (DNR) orders; (2) hospital policies should recognize the need for balanced protection of the patients and respect the right of a competent patient to make an informed choice; and (3) hospital policies should provide a means for appropriate resolution of conflicts and also mandate internal review. In addition to these broad guidelines, the report noted that much of medical practice is now governed by private and independent organizations, such as the Joint Commission on Accreditation of Healthcare Organizations (JCAHO), that bear a responsibility to encourage sound decisions regarding resuscitation. The President's Commission specifically suggested that, to be accredited, hospitals should be required to have at least a general policy regarding resuscitation, preferably one that addresses the three points cited above.

In response to these recommendations, as well as those from other health care organizations such as the American Hospital Association and the American Medical Association, the JCAHO did a survey of DNR policies in 1986. The purpose of this study was to determine the extent of use, nature, and implementation of DNR policies. Additional data identified common problems encountered in implementing DNR policies in addition to methods of resolving conflicts in the use of DNR orders. Enck et al. (1988) reported the clinically relevant results of this 1986 study, with a special comparative analysis of the hospice data.

A cross-sectional, random sample of health care organizations stratified by setting (acute care hospitals, psychiatric hospitals, long-term care facilities, hospices) were identified. A mail survey questionnaire was then sent to these 2,021 health care organizations; a response rate of 61 percent was obtained, with a confidence interval of 95 percent. The hospice sample size was 504, with a 62 percent response rate (312 hospices).

Overall, the results revealed variability across all settings in the extent of having formal, informal, or no DNR policies: 31 percent had a formal policy, 28 percent had an informal policy, and 41 percent had no policy. Hospices ranked second to acute care hospitals in having formal DNR policies (43% and 57%, respectively) (table 13.1).

In those hospices with a formal policy, DNR orders were written most often (90%) for patients with cancer, followed, in decreasing frequency, by patients with renal failure, stroke, congestive heart failure, Alzheimer disease and related disorders, coronary artery disease, acute myocardial infarction, and pneumonia.

If a decision was made for no cardiopulmonary resuscitation (CPR), defibrillation, intubation/ventilation, and medication were allowed in 69 percent of hospices and 79 percent of other settings with a formal DNR policy. Thus, in more than half of the hospices with a formal DNR policy, resuscitation measures other than CPR were included in the policy.

Table 13.1 Do-Not-Resuscitate (DNR) Treatment Policy, by Health Care Setting

Health Care Setting	Policy (%)		
	Formal	Informal	None
Acute care	57	9	14
Hospice care	43	20	7
Long-term care	20	30	50
Psychiatric care	11	8	80
Total (all settings)	31	28	41

Source: Enck et al. (1988).

Table 13.2   The Frequency of Common Problems Encountered in Implementing Do-Not-Resuscitate (DNR) Policies

Problem	Frequency (%)
Need for continuing education on this topic for nursing and medical staffs	41
Defining relationships of DNR to other treatments	38
Conflict between nursing and medical staffs as to appropriateness of DNR orders	33
Obtaining medical staff agreement/compliance with DNR policies	27
Legal issues	26
Obtaining attending physician countersignature in required time frame	24
Inability to establish functioning ethics/DNR related committee	18
Difficulty getting nursing staff to accept policies	10

Source: Enck et al. (1988).

Approximately one-fourth of hospices with a formal DNR policy addressed the withholding and/or withdrawal of treatments and interventions other than CPR. Hospices lacking a formal DNR policy, however, addressed these areas much less often (14%). Generally, in both groups these policies were in the following clinical areas: use of ventilator, nutrition/hydration, antibiotic therapy, and care of compromised infants.

In hospices with either formal, written DNR policies or informal, implicit policies, the need for continuing education on this topic for nursing and medical staffs was the most common problem of implementation. It was striking that one-third of the respondents reported nursing and medical staff conflict as a problem (table 13.2).

If conflicts in the use of DNR orders arose, resolution most often occurred by an informal meeting with family/guardian (68%). The use of the judicial system was the lowest-rated mechanism for resolving conflict (8%). Also, the conflict resolution process generally used a consultant for a second opinion regarding a patient's treatment or prognosis. In more than 90 percent of the responses, physicians in an appropriate specialty were identified as the consultants, followed by a nursing representative, clergy/spiritual counselor, medical director of a special unit, psychosocial worker, attorney, chief of staff, patient advocate, and ethicist/philosopher.

The ideal of providing maximal comfort to the dying patient through all phases of the terminal illness is a cornerstone of hospice care. Therefore, the investigators were surprised to find that only 43 percent of the hospices surveyed had a formal written policy on DNR. Furthermore, only one in five hospices had an informal policy, and more than one-third had no policy on DNR at all. On the other hand, hospices with a formal policy more clearly reflected the relationship of DNR to the patient's overall management than did acute, psychiatric, and long-term care settings. This critical insight into the complex role of DNR in patient care further strengthens the need for hospices to go through the process of developing these DNR policies, noted the authors.

As defined by Evans and Brody (1985), efforts at resuscitation may be divided into three categories: all available life-sustaining measures, all such measures except intubation, and basic CPR without active medications and intubation. In their study of three teaching hospitals, they reported that less than full efforts at resuscitation were made in 43 percent of cases where a final decision to resuscitate had not been made.

In an effort to further delineate the resuscitation efforts in hospice care, Enck et al. (1988) inquired about the use of other resuscitation measures (namely, defibrillation, intubation/ventilation, and chemical treatment) with patients when basic CPR was not performed. More than half allowed the use of these therapeutic interventions as part of a formal DNR policy, thus extending the observation of Evans and Brody (1985) that the DNR decision in the clinical setting is more often broad than it is narrow in scope.

Hospices with a formal DNR policy addressed the areas of withholding and/or withdrawing treatments more often than hospices without such formal policies. The use of a ventilator and nutrition/hydration were commonly cited clinical areas. Thus, those programs that went through the DNR decision-making process were also able to extend this into other areas, such as withholding or stopping interventions other than CPR (Enck et al. 1988).

In addressing the issue of survival of cancer patients after CPR, Faber-Langendoen (1991) reviewed all studies published from 1980 to 1989 that reported survival after CPR. Nine of these studies specifically included data on patients with cancer, and not all studies separated patients with metastatic cancer from those with localized disease. Fewer patients (3%) with cancer survived to hospital discharge than did patients with other diseases (12%). Of these survivors, all had localized disease. There were no survivors in any study among patients with metastatic cancer. In discussing these findings, Faber-Langendoen (1991) noted that, although communication and patient autonomy are critically important, physicians must not propose treatments that do not work, and CPR does not work for patients with metastatic cancer.

Indeed, not only patient communication and autonomy but also having the correct diagnosis of terminal cancer is of utmost importance. To this end, Rees, Dover, and Low-Beer (1987) reported the misdiagnosis of terminal cancer in four patients referred for supportive care. For a variety of reasons, each of these patients was wrongly labeled as having cancer when, in fact, nonmalignant diseases accounted for their failing health. When appropriately treated, they lived 18 months to 6+ years.

To identify the wishes of patients for information, participation in decision making, and life-sustaining treatment as well as to determine whether these wishes are stable over time, Silverstein et al. (1991) conducted a prospective survey of 38 patients with an established diagnosis of amyotrophic lateral sclerosis (ALS) at the University of Chicago Motor Neuron Disease Clinic. A baseline survey was done, and then the survey was repeated at six-month intervals. The interview format was used with a structured questionnaire. Twenty-five men and 13 women with an average age of 54 years participated in the study. The investigators found that preferences for CPR in two hypothetical circumstances, involving pneumonia, mechanical ventilation, and cardiac arrest, were much less stable over time than were desires for information and participation in decision making. Some patients changed their wishes from not wanting CPR to wanting it, whereas other patients changed their mind and no longer wanted to be resuscitated. Changes were not related to the patients' clinical or demographic characteristics. The authors concluded that, because many patients with ALS change their desire for life-sustaining treatment, advance directives for end-of-life care must be reevaluated periodically.

In a related study, Chochinov et al. (1999) examined the issue of the will to live in 168 terminally ill cancer patients, aged 31 to 89 years. The mean survival of these patients was 18 days. Twice daily the patients rated themselves on 100-point scales measuring pain, nausea, appetite, activity, drowsiness, sense of well-being, depression, anxiety, dyspnea, and the strength of their will to live. The authors found that the will to live was highly unstable among terminally ill cancer patients. This variation in the will to live changed as death neared. Initially, anxiety was the most significant predictor of the will to live. Subsequently, depression replaced anxiety, and in the final stages dyspnea was the most important variable. As death approached, the predominance of the psychological determinants of the will to live was replaced by the elements of physical distress as primary determinants. This substantial fluctuation in the will to live may alter a patient's decision-making process on life-sustaining treatments depending on the impact of psychological or physical distress.

Organizations such as the American Medical Association have provided guidelines for the appropriate use of DNR orders (Council on Ethical and Judicial Affairs 1991), which urge that these decisions be made openly. In an accompanying editorial, Lo (1991) offered some suggestions that may be helpful for physicians and patients in discussions about DNR orders. First, physicians should raise the subject of DNR in a straightforward manner and explain what CPR involves. Second, physicians must provide enough information for patients to make informed decisions. This discussion can be explicit without being threatening. Third, physicians should offer specific recommendations but also give the patient appropriate choices. Fourth, physicians should place CPR discussions in a positive context of supportive care while allaying patients' fear of pain and abandonment. Fifth, discussions about CPR need to be repeated, allowing the patients and families enough time to think about the issues and to deal with their emotions. And sixth, physicians can improve their skill at discussing DNR orders.

In 1995, the Study to Understand Prognoses and Preferences for Outcomes and Risks of Treatments (SUPPORT) (SUPPORT Principal Investigators 1995) demonstrated that most physicians did not know their patients' preferences regarding DNR orders. This landmark study demonstrated the lack of communication between physicians and their seriously ill patients about end-of-life issues. Eliasson et al. (1999) investigated the reasons why physicians did not write DNR orders when inpatients were faced with life-threatening situations. They found the major obstacle to be limitations in the length and depth of the patient-physician relationship. Moral objections to DNR orders, discomfort in discussing end-of-life issues, and the threat of litigation did not play a role. This study adds another point to Lo's (1991) suggestions, namely, that a conscious improvement in communication between physicians and patients is necessary.

Advance Directives

The Patient Self-Determination Act (PSDA), which went into effect in 1991, dictates that, as a requirement for Medicare and Medicaid payment, hospitals, skilled nursing facilities, home health agencies, hospices, and health maintenance organizations must do the following:

- develop written policies regarding advance directives;
- ask all new patients whether they have prepared an advance directive, such as a living will or durable power of attorney, and include this information on the patient's chart;
- give patients written materials regarding the institution's policies on advance directives and the patient's rights (under applicable state law) to prepare such documents; and
- educate the community and the institutional staff regarding advance directives (Greco et al. 1991).

Wolf et al. (1991) voiced concern that advance directives may wrongly be viewed as the only way to make future treatment decisions and may, furthermore, reduce the discussion of therapeutic alternatives and directives to a bureaucratic process dominated by forms and brochures. The authors emphasized the importance of periodic review of advance directives and thought that the PSDA's requirement should be seen as a catalyst for broader innovation to integrate advance directives into good patient care.

Enacting the PSDA, however, does not ensure that all adults will prepare or periodically update advance directives before a catastrophic illness. In this instance, there is often strong societal pressure in favor of preserving life regardless of the prognosis for recovery. Therefore, in many cases, the absence of an advance directive results in an implicit decision to start or continue life-sustaining treatment. This societal standard, however, conflicts with a growing body of evidence that most people do not want life-sustaining treatment if they become permanently unconscious or terminally ill. One possible solution to this dilemma would be for health care facilities to develop formal treatment guidelines based on the consensus of the lay and medical communities (Greco et al. 1991).

Ewer and Taubert (1995) prospectively studied 26 patients with cancer with advanced directives who were admitted to the intensive care unit of a major cancer hospital. Twenty-four of the 26 patients required mechanical ventilation. Eight patients died while on the ventilator, nine were terminally weaned, and seven were weaned and lived for at least 24 hours. Of these seven patients, six died before hospital discharge and one was discharged home. The most frequent problems encountered were the following:

- delay in presenting the advance directive;
- conflict between the dictates of the living will and the wishes of the person named in the durable power of attorney; and
- controversy among health care providers as to when in the course of the disease the spirit of the advanced directive had been met.

The authors concluded that considerable controversy exists regarding advance directives, and such documents often leave room for confusion regarding patients' desires in particular clinical situations.

Since the introduction of advance directives some 10 years ago, many unresolved problems remain. Although patients and health care providers express positive attitudes toward advance directives, they seldom complete the forms, and research efforts have increased the use of advance directives only modestly. Finally, advance preferences for treatment have been shown to be difficult to formulate, communicate, and implement (Martin, Emanuel, and Singer 2000).

The withdrawal of nutrition and hydration remains a controversial issue. Some are critical of stopping this form of treatment, which is considered a basic link between one person and another. The withdrawal of nutrition and hydration may also be perceived as directly hastening the death of a patient (Duffy 1992). In this particular matter, advance directives may not be helpful because of quirks of state law. Under Illinois law, for example, living wills do not apply to the withdrawal of nutrition and hydration (Blum 1990). However, in general the legal aspects of patients' requests for withdrawing or withholding life-sustaining treatment seem settled. No reported case has held a physician liable for complying with the wishes of the patient (Gostin 1997). Indeed, most court cases have not distinguished between withdrawing and withholding treatment (Rhymes et al. 2000).

Physician-Assisted Suicide and Euthanasia

The issue of a physician hastening a patient's death, be it actively (euthanasia) or passively (assisted suicide), is not new but has become very topical due to the publicity generated by the Michigan pathologist Dr. Jack Kevorkian (Enck 1999). The difference between physician-assisted suicide (PAS) and euthanasia is not really splitting hairs. By definition, PAS occurs when a physician provides the means or information for a person to perform the act to end his or her life. For example, if a physician gives a patient a prescription for sleeping pills and instructions on the fatal dosage and the patient takes the pills and dies, this is deemed physician-assisted suicide. On the other hand, euthanasia is when the physician actually performs the act that ends the patient's life. Dr. Kevorkian's injecting the lethal dose of Seconal into Mr. Youk's vein which resulted in his death is clearly euthanasia. The distinction between PAS and euthanasia is not superficial, because there are important legal ramifications. A physician who commits euthanasia may be criminally charged with murder, as in the case of Dr. Kevorkian, whereas a physician who assists in a patient's suicide can be criminally charged under existing laws in 25 states with a felony less serious than homicide (Stone and Winslade 1995).

Since 1950, there have been seven cases of physicians prosecuted for murder after euthanasia. An illustrative case is that of Dr. Joseph Hassman, who in 1986 was charged with manslaughter after injecting his mother-in-law with a lethal dose of Demerol. Dr. Hassman pleaded guilty and was given two years of probation. Dr. Kevorkian's conviction in 1999 of second-degree murder was the first time a jury had found a physician guilty of homicide. In contrast, no physician has been convicted for physician-assisted suicide, including the highly publicized Dr. Timothy Quill (Stone and Winslade 1995). Dr. Quill, who wrote of his experience in the *New England Journal of Medicine* (Quill 1991), was charged under New York State's assisted suicide laws for the death of his patient, Patricia Diane Trumbull. A grand jury, however, refused to indict Dr. Quill. This failure to indict Dr. Quill and others reflects growing public support for physician-assisted suicide.

Surveys suggest that about two-thirds of Americans favor legalization of physician-assisted suicide (Bachman et al. 1996; Churchill and King 1997). However, this sentiment may not mirror reality, since legalization of assisted suicide has been introduced and defeated in the states of Washington (1991), California (1992), and Michigan (1998). The Oregon Death with Dignity Act was passed in a statewide referendum by a narrow margin in 1994 but was never enacted due to legal obstacles. In 1997, it was placed back on the ballot and was overwhelmingly passed again.

Unlike the general public, the majority of physicians oppose PAS (Council on Scientific Affairs 1996). The societal issue of the "slippery slope" is often stated as an objection. In essence, this is the concern that the legalization of PAS will gradually extend to include those patients not terminally ill but a burden to society, in addition to the expansion of physician activities to euthanasia (Churchill and King 1997). However, as pointed out by Angell (1997), fears of the "slippery slope" have not been borne out in the Netherlands, where both physician-assisted suicide and euthanasia are permitted under law. Furthermore, as suggested by Quill, Lee, and Nunn (2000), a covert practice of PAS exists in the United States.

On October 27, 1998, Oregon became the first state to legalize physician-assisted suicide with the Oregon Death with Dignity Act. This act enables terminally ill state residents to receive prescriptions of self-administered lethal medications from their physicians, but does not permit euthanasia. The law has strict guidelines and stipulates that the Oregon resident must be able to make and communicate decisions about his or her health care and must have an illness with six months or less survival. The patient must make one written and two oral requests to his or her physician, and the oral requests must be separated by at least 15 days. Confirmation of the diagnosis of a terminal disease and the prognosis, determination that the patient is able to make decisions, and referral for counseling if there is some doubt whether the patient's judgment is impaired by psychological disorder are required by the patient's primary physician and a consultant. The primary physician must inform the patient of all alternatives, such as comfort care, hospice, and pain-control options. Finally, to comply with the law, physicians must report all prescriptions they write to the Oregon Health Division.

Given the above constraints on PAS, the publication of Oregon's first-year experience with legalized PAS is most interesting (Chin et al. 1999). Twenty-three patients requested prescriptions for lethal drugs, and 15 died after taking the medication, 6 died from the underlying disease, and 2 were alive as of January 1, 1999. The median age of the 15 patients who died from lethal medication was 69 years, with 8 being male and all 15 being white. Thirteen of the 15 had cancer. With one exception, the prescriptions were for 9 g of a fast-acting barbiturate (secobarbital or pentobarbital) and an antiemetic. Although most patients died within 1 hour, four died within 3 hours of taking the drugs and one died 11.5 hours later.

Chin et al. (1999) addressed the important question of patients requesting PAS because of inadequate care at the end of life. The authors thought, based on the data, that this was not the case. Ten of the 15 patients (71%) were enrolled in a hospice program, which is not surprising, since Oregon ranks third nationally in the rate of admission to hospice. Only 1 of the 15 patients expressed concern about inadequate pain control at the end of life. Loss of autonomy and loss of control of bodily functions were the major reasons for patients requesting PAS. Seventy-nine percent of the patients were not completely disabled when they took the lethal medications, which suggests, according to the authors, that controlling the time of death was important to them. The authors concluded that, during the first year of legalized PAS in Oregon, a patient's decision to request and use a prescription of lethal medications was associated with concern about loss of autonomy or control of bodily functions, not a fear of intractable pain or worries about financial loss. A subsequent publication on the second year of experience in Oregon (Sullivan, Hedberg, and Fleming 2000) confirmed these findings and reaffirmed the importance of patients' control over how they die.

In contrast to the popular belief that most terminally ill patients desire PAS to avoid dying in excruciating, uncontrolled pain, the Oregon experience suggests otherwise. Emanuel and Emanuel (1998) reached the same conclusion, that is, that pain is not a major factor motivating requests for PAS or euthanasia. Furthermore, they reported that patients who are depressed, have other psychological distress, or have significant caregiver difficulties are more likely to desire PAS or euthanasia. By comparison, only 4 of the 15 patients (27%) in the Oregon study (Chin et al. 1999) were referred for psychiatric or psychological counseling as required by law. This implies that depression does not play a major role in patients seeking PAS. More insight into this issue is provided by a study of patients with amyotrophic lateral sclerosis (ALS). Ganzini et al. (1998) surveyed 100 patients with ALS and their families in Oregon and Washington state to determine their attitudes toward PAS. They reported that the majority of patients would consider PAS and that many would request a prescription for lethal medication well before they intended to use it.

They found that hopelessness, but not depression, was associated with a desire to consider PAS.

Like any other medical procedure, PAS and euthanasia are subject to untoward events. Groenewoud et al. (2000) reported on clinical problems occurring with PAS and euthanasia in the Netherlands, where both are legal. Complications such as myoclonus, cyanosis, nausea, and vomiting occurred in 7 percent of the cases of assisted suicide. Problems with completion of the suicide, mainly longer time to death than expected and failure to induce coma, were noted in 16 percent of the patients. Complications and problems with completion happened less often in cases of euthanasia: 3 percent and 6 percent, respectively. In 18 percent of the cases, assisted suicide became euthanasia because of the patient's inability to take the medication or problems with the completion of the PAS.

These recent scientific studies provide some insight into PAS and euthanasia and the reasons why patients seek this method to end their lives. Clinically relevant observations include the following:

- the fear of terminal, intractable pain is not a major factor in patients pursuing PAS;
- the popular view of a depressed, dying patient seeking PAS may not be accurate;
- recognition of hopeless feelings in patients is important, and they must be addressed;
- it is critical that the physician deal with the patient's perception of loss of autonomy and personal freedom as his or her life nears the end;
- clinicians must pay more attention to actively managing the loss of bodily functions that are of concern to dying patients; and
- physician-assisted suicide is not without clinical complications and problems.

Summary

Hospices and other health care organizations caring for dying patients need to develop formal DNR policies, since this decision-making process is easily extended into other areas, such as withholding or stopping interventions other than CPR. The importance of addressing the DNR issue is highlighted by a study (Faber-Langendoen 1991) that found no survivors after CPR in patients with metastatic cancer. On the other hand, before a DNR decision is made regarding a terminally ill cancer patient, the diagnosis must be correct (Rees, Dover, and Low-Beer 1987). Critical to making a DNR order is a frank and open discussion between the patient and the physician. This discussion should be repeated periodically, since some patients change their minds, as noted in patients with ALS (Silverstein et al. 1991) and advanced cancer (Chochinov et al. 1999).

Although advance directives are a requirement for Medicare and Medicaid reimbursement, controversy still exists regarding their formulation and implementation (Ewer and Taubert 1995; Martin, Emanuel, and Singer 2000). Legally, the issue of patients' requests for withdrawing or withholding life-sustaining treatment seems settled (Gostin 1997). However, clinical uncertainty and debate continue on these important issues. Finally, the fear of intractable terminal pain is not a major factor in patients seeking physician-assisted suicide, but PAS is not without significant clinical complications and problems (Groenewoud et al. 2000).

References

Abrahm, J. L. 1999. Management of pain and spinal cord compression in patients with advanced cancer. *Annals of Internal Medicine* 131:37–46.

Abrahm, J. L. 2000. *A Physician's Guide to Pain and Symptom Management in Cancer Patients.* Baltimore: Johns Hopkins University Press.

Acute Pain Management Guideline Panel. 1992. Options to prevent and control postoperative pain. In *Acute Pain Management: Operative or Medical Procedures and Trauma. Clinical Practice Guideline,* 15–26. Rockville, Md.: Agency for Health Care Policy and Research, Public Health Service, U. S. Department of Health and Human Services.

Adam, J. 1997. The last 48 hours. *British Medical Journal* 315:1600–1603.

Ahlquist, D. A., C. J. Gostout, T. R. Viggiano, R. K. Balm, P. C. Pairolero, V. S. Hench, and A. R. Zinsmeister. 1987. Endoscopic laser palliation of malignant dysphagia: A prospective study. *Mayo Clinic Proceedings* 62:867–74.

Ahmedzai, S., and D. Brooks. 1997. Transdermal fentanyl versus sustained-release oral morphine in cancer pain: Preference, efficacy, and quality of life. *Journal of Pain and Symptom Management* 13:254–61.

Allan, S. G. 1988. Emesis in the patient with advanced cancer. *Palliative Medicine* 2:89–100.

Allman, R. M. 1989. Pressure ulcers among the elderly. *New England Journal of Medicine* 320:850–53.

Allman, R. M., C. L. Laprade, L. B. Noel, J. M. Walker, C. A. Moorer, M. R. Dear, and C. R. Smith. 1986. Pressure sores among hospitalized patients. *Annals of Internal Medicine* 105:337- 42.

Allman, R. M., J. M. Walker, M. K. Hart, C. A. Laprade, L. B. Noel, and C. R. Smith. 1987. Air-fluidized beds or conventional therapy for pressure sores. *Annals of Internal Medicine* 107:641–48.

American College of Physicians. 1989. Parenteral nutrition in patients receiving cancer chemotherapy. *Annals of Internal Medicine* 110:734–36.

Amesbury, B. D. W., and K. P. Dunphy. 1989. The use of subcutaneous midazolam in the home care setting. *Palliative Medicine* 3:299–301.

Andrews, M. R., and A. M. Levine. 1989. Dehydration in the terminal patient: Perception of hospice nurses. *American Journal of Hospice Care* 6:31–34.

Angell, M. 1982. The quality of mercy. *New England Journal of Medicine* 306:98–99.

Angell, M. 1997. The Supreme Court and physician-assisted suicide—the ultimate right. *New England Journal of Medicine* 336:50–53.

Aranha, G. V., F. A. Folk, and H. B. Greenlee. 1981. Surgical palliation of small bowel obstruction due to metastatic cancer. *American Surgeon* 47:99–102.

Ashby, M., and B. Stoffell. 1991. Therapeutic ratio and defined phases: Proposal of ethical framework for palliative care. *British Medical Journal* 302:1322–24.

Ashford, R., G. Plant, J. Maher, and L. Teare. 1984. Double-blind trial of metronidazole in malodorous ulcerating tumors. *Lancet* 1:1232–33.

Avellanosa, A. M., and C. R. West. 1982. Experience with transcutaneous nerve stimulation for relief of intractable pain in cancer patients. *Journal of Medicine* 13:203–13.

Bachman, J. G., K. H. Alcser, D. J. Doukas, R. L. Lichtenstein, A. D. Corning, and H. Brody. 1996. Attitudes of Michigan physicians and the public toward legalizing physician-assisted suicide and voluntary euthanasia. *New England Journal of Medicine* 334:303–9.

Backonja, M., A. Beydoun, K. R. Edwards, S. L. Schwartz, V. Fonseca, M. Hes, L. LaMoreaux, and E. Garofalo. 1998. Gabapentin for the symptomatic treatment of painful neuropathy in patients with diabetes mellitus: A randomized controlled trial. *Journal of the American Medical Association* 280:1831–36.

Baines, M., D. J. Oliver, and R. L. Carter. 1985. Medical management of intestinal obstruction in patients with advanced malignant disease: A clinical and pathological study. *Lancet* 2:990–93.

Baines, M. J. 1997. Nausea and vomiting. *British Medical Journal* 315:1148–50.

Baker, A. R. 1989. Treatment of malignant ascites. In *Cancer: Principles and Practice of Oncology,* ed. V. T. DeVita, S. Hellman, and S. A. Rosenberg, chapter 62, section 6. Philadelphia: J. B. Lippincott.

Bale, S., and C. Regnard. 1989. Pressure sores in advanced disease: A flow diagram. *Palliative Medicine* 3:263–65.

Barr, H., and N. Krasner. 1991. Prospective quality of life analysis after palliative photoablation for the treatment of malignant dysphagia. *Cancer* 68:1660–64.

Baumrucker, S. J. 1998. Management of intestinal obstruction in hospice care. *American Journal of Hospice and Palliative Care* 15:232–35.

Bell, M. D. D., P. Mishra, B. D. Weldon, G. R. Murray, T. N. Calvey, and N. E. Williams. 1985. Buccal morphine: A new route for analgesia? *Lancet* 1:71–73.

Berger, J. M., A. Ryan, N. Vadivelu, P. Merriam, L. Rever, and P. Harrison. 2000. Ketamine-fentanyl-midazolam infusion for the control of symptoms in terminal life care. *American Journal of Hospice and Palliative Care* 17:127–32.

Bergner, M., L. D. Hudson, D. A. Conrad, C. M. Patmont, G. J. McDonald, E. B. Perrin, and B. S. Gibson. 1988. The cost and efficacy of home care for patients with chronic lung disease. *Medical Care* 26:566–79.

Bernabei, R., G. Gambassi, K. Lapane, F. Landi, C. Gatsonis, R. Dunlop, L. Lipsitz, K. Steel, and V. Mor. 1998. Mangement of pain in elderly patients with cancer. *Journal of the American Medical Association* 279:1877–82.

Berry, J. I. 1988. The use of analgesics in patients with pain from terminal disease. *American Journal of Hospice Care* 5:26–42.

Block, S. D. 2000. Assessing and managing depression in the terminally ill patient. *Annals of Internal Medicine* 132:209–18.

Blum, J. D. 1990. The legal dilemma of stopping artificial feeding. *American Journal of Hospice and Palliative Care* 7:42–48.

Bono, B., P. Cazzaniga, V. Pini, S. M. Zurrida, R. Spagnolo, L. Torelli, C. Corona, and A. Bono. 1991. Palliative surgery of metastatic bone disease: A review of 83 cases. *European Journal of Cancer* 27:556–58.

Brechling, B. G., and D. Kuhn. 1989. A specialized hospice for dementia patients and their families. *American Journal of Hospice Care* 6:27–30.

Breitbart, W. 1987. Suicide in cancer patients. *Oncology* 1:49–54.

Brown, J. H., P. Henteleff, S. Barakat, and C. J. Rowe. 1986. Is it normal for terminally ill patients to desire death? *American Journal of Psychiatry* 143:208–11.

Brozena, S. 1999. End-stage heart failure: Palliation and terminal care. *Wissahickon Hospice Physician Update* Spring:1–2.

Bruera, E., and N. MacDonald. 1986. Intractable pain in patients with advanced head and neck tumors: A possible role of local infection. *Cancer Treatment Reports* 70:691–92.

Bruera, E., and N. MacDonald. 2000. To hydrate or not to hydrate: How should it be? *Journal of Clinical Oncology* 18:1156–58.

Bruera E., E. Roca, L. Cedaro, S. Carraro, and R. Chacon. 1985. Action of oral methylprednisolone in terminal cancer patients: A prospective randomized double-blind study. *Cancer Treatment Reports* 69:751–54.

Bruera, E., S. Carraro, E. Roca, M. Barugel, and R. Chacon. 1986a. Double-blind evaluation of the effects of mazindol on pain, depression, anxiety, appetite, and activity in terminal cancer patients. *Cancer Treatment Reports* 70:295–98.

Bruera, E., S. Chadwick, R. Fox, J. Hanson, and N. MacDonald. 1986b. Study of cardiovascular autonomic insufficiency in advanced cancer patients. *Cancer Treatment Reports* 70:1383–87.

Bruera, E., C. Brenneis, M. Michaud, and N. MacDonald. 1987a. Continuous SC infusion of metoclopramede for treatment of narcotic bowel syndrome. *Cancer Treatment Reports* 71:1121–22.

Bruera, E., S. Chadwick, A. Weinlick, and N. MacDonald. 1987b. Delirium and severe sedation in patients with terminal cancer. *Cancer Treatment Reports* 71:787–88.

Bruera, E., C. Brenneis, M. Michaud, S. Chadwick, and N. MacDonald. 1987c. Continuous SC infusion of narcotics using a portable disposable device in patients with advanced cancer. *Cancer Treatment Reports* 71:635–37.

Bruera, E., S. Chadwick, C. Brenneis, J. Hanson, and N. MacDonald. 1987d. Methylphenidate associated with narcotics for the treatment of cancer pain. *Cancer Treatment Reports* 71:67–70.

Bruera, E., C. Brenneis, M. Michaud, P. I. Jackson, and R. N. MacDonald. 1988a. Muscle electrophysiology in patients with advanced breast cancer. *Journal of the National Cancer Institute* 80:282–85.

Bruera, E., C. Brenneis, M. Michaud, R. Bacovsky, S. Chadwick, A. Emeno, and N. MacDonald. 1988b. Use of the subcutaneous route for the administration of narcotics in patients with cancer pain. *Cancer* 62:407–11.

Bruera, E., M. A. Legris, N. Kuehn, and M. J. Miller. 1990. Hypodermoclysis for the administration of fluids and narcotic analgesics in patients with advanced cancer. *Journal of Pain and Symptom Management* 5:218–20.

Bruera, E., N. de Stoutz, A. Velasco-Leiva, T. Schoeller, and J. Hanson. 1993. Effects of oxygen on dyspnoea in hypoxaemic terminal-cancer patients. *Lancet* 342:13–14.

Bruera, E., R. Fainsinger, K. Spachynski, N. Babul, Z. Harsanyi, and A. C. Darke. 1995. Clinical efficacy and safety of a novel controlled-release morphine suppository and subcutaneous morphine in cancer pain: A randomized evaluation. *Journal of Clinical Oncology* 13:1520–27.

Bruera, E., M. Belzile, E. Pituskin, R. Fainsinger, A. Darke, Z. Harsanyi, N. Babul, and I. Ford. 1998. Randomized, double-blind, cross-over trial comparing safety and efficacy of oral controlled-release morphine in patients with cancer pain. *Journal of Clinical Oncology* 16:3222–29.

Brusis, T., and H. Luckhaupt. 1989. Fetor from ulcerated head and neck tumors: Causation and therapy. *Annals of Otology, Rhinology and Laryngology* 98:615–17.

Bunn, P. A., and E. C. Ridgway. 1989. Paraneoplastic syndromes. In *Cancer: Principles and Practice of Oncology,* ed. V. T. DeVita, S. Hellman, and S. A. Rosenberg, chapter 55. Philadelphia: J. B. Lippincott.

Caplan, R. A., L. B. Ready, R. V. Oden, F. A. Matsen, M. L. Nessly, and G. L. Olsson. 1989. Transdermal fentanyl for postoperative pain management: A double-blind placebo study. *Journal of the American Medical Association* 260: 1036–39.

Carlson, R. W., L. Devich, and R. R. Frank. 1988. Development of a comprehensive support care team for the hopelessly ill on a university hospital medical service. *Journal of the American Medical Association* 259:378–83.

Carter, R. L., M. R. Pittam, and N. S. B. Tanner. 1982. Pain and dysphagia in patients with squamous carcinomas of the head and neck: The role of perineural spread. *Journal of the Royal Society of Medicine* 75:598–606.

Cassileth, B. R. 1999. Complementary and alternative cancer medicine. *Journal of Clinical Oncology* 17 (November Supplement):44–52.

Chang, V. T. 2000. The value of symptoms in prognosis of cancer patients. In *Topics in Palliative Care,* ed. R. K. Portenoy and E. Bruera, chapter 2. New York: Oxford University Press.

Chapman, C. R., and H. F. Hill. 1989. Prolonged morphine self-administration and addiction liability: Evaluation of two theories in a bone marrow transplantation unit. *Cancer* 63:1636–44.

Chatal, J. F., and C. A. Hoefnagel. 1999. Nuclear medicine: Radionuclide therapy. *Lancet* 354:931–35.

Cherny, N. I. 2000. The use of sedation in the management of refractory pain. *Principles and Practice of Supportive Oncology Updates* 3:1–11.

Cherny, N. I., and K. M. Foley. 1996. Nonopioid and opioid analgesic pharmacotherapy of cancer pain. *Hematology/Oncology Clinics of North America* 10:79–102.

Chin, A. E., K. Hedberg, G. K. Higginson, and D. W. Fleming. 1999. Legalized physician-assisted suicide in Oregon—The first year's experience. *New England Journal of Medicine* 340:577–83.

Chochinov, H. M., D. Tataryn, J. J. Clinch, and D. Dudgeon. 1999. Will to live in the terminally ill. *Lancet* 354:816–19.

Christakis, N. A., and E. B. Lamont. 2000. Extent and determinants of error in doctors' prognoses in terminally ill patients: Prospective cohort study. *British Medical Journal* 320:469–72.

Christie, J. M., M. Simmonds, R. Patt, P. Coluzzi, M. A. Busch, E. Nordbrock, and

R. K. Portenoy. 1998. Dose-titration, multicenter study of oral transmucosal fentanyl citrate for the treatment of breakthrough pain in cancer patients using transdermal fentanyl for persistent pain. *Journal of Clinical Oncology* 16: 3238–45.

Churchill, L. R., and N. M. P. King. 1997. Physician assisted suicide, euthanasia, or withdrawal of treatment. *British Medical Journal* 315:137–38.

Citron, M. L., A. Johnston-Early, M. Boyer, S. H. Krasnow, M. Hood, and M. H. Cohen. 1986. Patient-controlled analgesic for severe cancer pain. *Archives of Internal Medicine* 146:734–36.

Clark, J. D., and T. Edwards. 1999. Severe respiratory depression in a patient with gastroparesis while receiving opioids for pain. *Clinical Journal of Pain* 15:321–23.

Clarke, C., I. McConachie, J. D. Edwards, and P. Nightingale. 1990. Concealed haemorrhage in patients nursed on an air-fluidised bed. *British Medical Journal* 301:432.

Cleeland, C. S., R. Gonin, A. K. Hatfield, J. H. Edmonson, R. H. Blum, J. A. Stewart, and K. J. Pandya. 1994. Pain and its treatment in outpatients with metastatic cancer. *New England Journal of Medicine* 330:592–96.

Cody, M. 1990. Depression and the use of antidepressants in patients with cancer. *Palliative Medicine* 4:271–78.

Colburn, L. 1987. Pressure ulceration prevention for the hospice patient. *American Journal of Hospice Care* 4:22–26.

Cole, R. M. 1991. Medical aspects of care for the person with advanced acquired immunodeficiency syndrome (AIDS): A palliative care perspective. *Palliative Medicine* 5:96–111.

Consensus Conference. 1989. Urinary incontinence in adults. *Journal of the American Medical Association* 261:2685–90.

Cooke, N. 1989. Dyspnea. In *Symptom Control*, ed. T. D. Walsh, chapter 14. Boston: Blackwell Scientific Publications.

Corcoran, C., and S. Grinspoon. 1999. Treatments for wasting in patients with the acquired immunodeficiency syndrome. *New England Journal of Medicine* 340: 1740–50.

Council on Ethical and Judicial Affairs. 1991. Guidelines for the appropriate use of do-not-resuscitate orders. *Journal of the American Medical Association* 265: 1868–71.

Council on Scientific Affairs. 1996. Good care of the dying patient. *Journal of the American Medical Association* 275:474–78.

Cousins, M. J., and L. E. Mather. 1984. Intrathecal and epidural administration of opioids. *Anesthesiology* 61:276–310.

Coyle, N., A. Mauskop, J. Maggard, and K. M. Foley. 1986. Continuous subcutaneous infusions of opiates in cancer patients with pain. *Oncology Nursing Forum* 13:53–57.

Coyle, N., J. Adelhardt, K. M. Foley, and R. K. Portenoy. 1990. Character of terminal illness in the advanced cancer patient: Pain and other symptoms during the last four weeks of life. *Journal of Pain and Symptom Management* 5:83–93.

Curtis, E. B., R. Krech, and T. D. Walsh. 1991. Common symptoms in patients with advanced cancer. *Journal of Palliative Care* 7:25–29.

Davis, C. L. 1997. Breathlessness, cough, and other respiratory problems. *British Medical Journal* 315:931–34.

De Conno, F. 1998. Adjuvant analgesics (co-analgesics). In *2nd International Conference 1998—Comprehensive Cancer Care (ICCC)*, ed. S. Kaasa, 7–8. Limassol, Cyprus: Hadjigeorgiou Printing and Co., Ltd.

De Conno, F., C. Ripamonti, L. Saita, T. MacEachern, J. Hanson, and E. Bruera. 1995. Role of rectal route in treating cancer pain: A randomized crossover clinical trial of oral versus rectal morphine administration in opioid-naïve cancer patients with pain. *Journal of Clinical Oncology* 13:1004–8.

Della Cuna, G. R., A. Pellegrini, and M. Piazzi. 1989. Effect of methylprednisolone sodium succinate on quality of life in preterminal cancer patients: A placebo-controlled, multicenter study. *European Journal of Cancer and Clinical Oncology* 25:1817–21.

Derogatis, L. R., and R. N. MacDonald. 1982. Psychopharmacologic applications to cancer. *Cancer* 50:1968–73.

Derogatis, L. R., G. R. Morrow, J. Fetting, D. Penman, S. Piasetsky, A. M. Schmale, M. Henrichs, and C. L. M. Carnicke. 1983. The prevalence of psychiatric disorders among cancer patients. *Journal of the American Medical Association* 249:751–57.

Devulder, J., L. Ghys, W. Dhondt, and G. Rolly. 1994. Spinal analgesia in terminal care: Risk versus benefit. *Journal of Pain and Symptom Management* 9:75–81.

DeWys, W. D., and F. A. Hoffman. 1984. Pathophysiology of anorexia and disturbances of taste in cancer patients. In *Frontiers in Gastrointestinal Cancer*, ed. B. Levin and R. H. Riddell, 81–90. New York: Elsevier.

DeWys, W. D., C. Begg, P. T. Lavin, P. R. Band, J. M. Bennett, J. R. Bertino, M. H. Cohen, H. O. Douglass, P. F. Engstrom, E. Z. Ezdinli, J. Horton, G. J. Johnson, C. G. Moertel, M. M. Oken, C. Perlia, C. Rosenbaum, M. N. Silverstein, R. T. Skeel, R. W. Sponzo, and D. C. Tormey. 1980. Prognostic effect of weight loss prior to chemotherapy in cancer patients. *American Journal of Medicine* 69:491–97.

Dodds, L. J. 1985. The control of cancer chemotherapy–induced nausea and vomiting. *Journal of Clinical and Hospital Pharmacy* 10:143–66.

Duffield, M. 1989. Bedsores. In *Symptom Control*, ed. T. D. Walsh, chapter 4. Boston: Blackwell Scientific Publications.

Duffy, T. P. 1992. Clinical problem-solving. *New England Journal of Medicine* 326:933–35.

DuPen, S. L., D. G. Peterson, A. C. Bogosian, D. H. Ramsey, C. Larson, and M. Omoto. 1987. A new permanent exteriorized epidural catheter for narcotic self-administration to control cancer pain. *Cancer* 59:986–93.

Duthie, D. J. R., and W. S. Nimmo. 1987. Adverse effects of opioid analgesic drugs. *British Journal of Anaesthesiology* 59:61–77.

Editorial. 1986a. Spinal opiates revisited. *Lancet* 1:655–56.

Editorial. 1986b. Terminal dehydration. *Lancet* 1:306.

Editorial. 1990a. Management of smelly tumours. *Lancet* 335:141–42.

Editorial. 1990b. Strontium and bone pain. *Lancet* 335:384–85.

Editorial. 1992. Endoprosthesis for bone metastases. *Lancet* 339:1145.

Eliasson, A. H., J. M. Parker, A. F. Shorr, K. A. Babb, R. Harris, B. A. Aaronson, and M. Diemer. 1999. Impediments to writing do-not-resuscitate orders. *Archives of Internal Medicine* 159:2213–18.

Ellison, N. M., and G. O. Lewis. 1984. Plasma concentrations following single doses of morphine sulfate in oral solution and rectal suppository. *Clinical Pharmacy* 3:614–17.

Emanuel, E. J., and L. L. Emanuel. 1998. The promise of a good death. *Lancet* 351(supp II):21–29.

Enck, R. E. 1991. Pain control in the ambulatory elderly. *Geriatrics* 46:49–60.

Enck, R. E. 1992. A review of pain management. *American Journal of Hospice and Palliative Care* 9:6–12.

Enck, R. E. 1995. Pain management and parenteral opioids: An update. *American Journal of Hospice and Palliative Care* 12:8–13.

Enck, R. E. 1999. Jack Kevorkian: "Too much. " *American Journal of Hospice and Palliative Medicine* 16:375–76.

Enck, R. E., D. R. Longa, M. W. Arren, and B. A. McCann. 1988. DNR policies in healthcare organizations with emphasis on hospice. *American Journal of Hospice Care* 5:39–42.

Ernst, E., and B. R. Cassileth. 1998. The prevalence of complementary/alternative medicine in cancer: A systematic review. *Cancer* 83:777–82.

Estenne, M., J. C. Yernault, and A. DeTroyer. 1983. Mechanism of relief of dyspnea after thoracocentesis in patients with large pleural effusions. *American Journal of Medicine* 74:813–19.

Evans, A. L., and B. A. Brody. 1985. The do-not-resuscitate order in teaching hospitals. *Journal of the American Medical Association* 253:2236–39.

Evans, C., and M. McCarthy. 1985. Prognostic uncertainty in terminal care: Can the Karnofsky index help? *Lancet* 1:1204–6.

Ewer, M. S., and J. K. Taubert. 1995. Advance directives in the intensive care unit of a tertiary cancer center. *Cancer* 76:1268–74.

Expert Working Group of the European Association for Palliative Care. Morphine in cancer pain: Modes of administration. 1996. *British Medical Journal* 312:823–26.

Faber-Langendoen, K. 1991. Resuscitation of patients with metastatic cancer: Is transient benefit still futile? *Archives of Internal Medicine* 151:235–39.

Fabiszewski, K. J., B. Volicer, and L. Volicer. 1990. Effect of antibiotic treatment on outcome of fevers in institutionalized Alzheimer patients. *Journal of the American Medical Association* 263:3168–72.

Fainsinger, R. L. 1998. Dehydration of the terminally ill. *American Journal of Hospice and Palliative Care* 15:255–56.

Fainsinger, R. L., and E. Bruera. 1991. Hypodermoclysis (HDC) for symptom control vs. the Edmonton Injector (EI). *Journal of Palliative Care* 7:5–8.

Fainsinger, R., M. J. Miller, E. Bruera, J. Hanson, and T. MacEachern. 1991. Symptom control during the last week of life on a palliative care unit. *Journal of Palliative Care* 7:5–11.

Fallon, M., and B. O'Neill. 1997. Constipation and diarrhoea. *British Medical Journal* 315:1293–96.

Farrar, J. T., J. Cleary, R. Rauck, M. Busch, and E. Nordbrock. 1998. Oral transmucosal fentanyl citrate: Randomized, double-blinded, placebo-controlled trial for treatment of breakthrough pain in cancer patients. *Journal of the National Cancer Institute* 90:611–16.

Ferrer-Brechner, T. 1989. Anesthetic techniques for the management of cancer pain. *Cancer* 63:2343–47.

Ferri, F. F. 1998. Infectious diseases. In *Practical Guide to the Care of the Medical Patient,* ed. F. F. Ferri, chapter 22. St. Louis: Mosby.

Ferris, F. D. 1990. Pre-terminal delirium. In *A Practical Seminar/Workshop on Narcotic Infusions,* ed. F. D. Ferris, 25–28. Toronto: Pain Management Group.

Filshie, J., and P. J. Morrison. 1988. Acupuncture for chronic pain: A review. *Palliative Medicine* 2:1–14.

Filshie, J., and D. Redman. 1985. Acupuncture and malignant pain problems. *European Journal of Surgical Oncology* 11:389–94.

Finlay, I. G. 1986. Oral symptoms and candida in the terminally ill. *British Medical Journal* 292:592–93.

Finucane, T. E., C. Christmas, and K. Travis. 1999. Tube feeding in patients with advanced dementia: A review of the evidence. *Journal of the American Medical Association* 282:1365–70.

Foley, K. 1999. A 44-year-old woman with severe pain at the end of life. *Journal of the American Medical Association* 281:1937–45.

Foley, K. M. 1985. The treatment of cancer pain. *New England Journal of Medicine* 313:84–95.

Foley, K. M. 1989. Controversies in cancer pain: Medical perspectives. *Cancer* 63:2257–65.

Foley, K. M., and E. Arbit. 1989. Management of cancer pain. In *Cancer: Principles and Practice of Oncology,* ed. V. T. DeVita, S. Hellman, and S. A. Rosenberg, chapter 59, section 4. Philadelphia: J. B. Lippincott.

Foley, K. M., and C. E. Inturrisi. 1987. Analgesic drug therapy in cancer pain: Principles and practice. *Medical Clinics of North America* 71:207–32.

Forbes, J. F. 1988. Principles and potential of palliative surgery in patients with advanced cancer. In: *Supportive Care in Cancer Patients,* ed. H. J. Senn, A. Glaus, and L. Schmid, 134–42. New York: Springer-Verlag.

Forrest, W. H., B. W. Brown, C. R. Brown, R. Defalque, M. Gold, H. E. Gordon, K. E. James, J. Katz, D. L. Mahler, P. Schroff, and G. Teutsch. 1977. Dextroamphetamine with morphine for the treatment of postoperative pain. *New England Journal of Medicine* 296:712–15.

Forster, L. E., and J. Lynn. 1988. Predicting life span for applicants to inpatient hospice. *Archives of Internal Medicine* 148:2540–43.

Forster, L. E., and J. Lynn. 1989. The use of physiologic measures and demographic variables to predict longevity among inpatient hospice applicants. *American Journal of Hospice Care* 6:31–34.

Fox, E., K. Landrum-McNiff, Z. Zhong, N. V. Dawson, A. W. Wu, and J. Lynn. 1999. Evaluation of prognostic criteria for determining hospice eligibility in patients with advanced lung, heart, or liver disease. *Journal of the American Medical Association* 282:1638–45.

Frytak, S., and C. G. Moertel. 1981. Management of nausea and vomiting in the cancer patient. *Journal of the American Medical Association* 245:393–96.

Ganzini, L., W. S. Johnston, B. H. McFarland, S. W. Tolle, and M. A. Lee. 1998. Attitudes of patients with amyotrophic lateral sclerosis and their care givers toward assisted suicide. *New England Journal of Medicine* 339:967–73.

Ghajar, J. 2000. Traumatic brain injury. *Lancet* 356:923–29.

Gibbs, L. M. E., J. Addington-Hall, and J. S. R. Gibbs. 1998. Dying from heart failure: Lessons from palliative care. *British Medical Journal* 317:961–62.

Gillick, M. R. 2000. Rethinking the role of tube feeding in patients with advanced dementia. *New England Journal of Medicine* 342:206–10.

Glass, R. M. 1983. Psychiatric disorders among cancer patients. *Journal of the American Medical Association* 249:782–83.

Gold, J. W. M. 1992. HIV-1 infection. Diagnosis and management. *Medical Clinics of North America* 76:1–18.

Gostin, L. O. 1997. Deciding life and death in the courtroom. *Journal of the American Medical Association* 278:1523–28.

Greco, P. J., K. A. Schulman, R. Lavizzo-Mourey, and J. Hansen-Flaschen. 1991. The Patient self-Determination Act and the future of advance directives. *Annals of Internal Medicine* 115:639–43.

Greene, W. R., and W. H. Davis. 1991. Titrated intravenous barbiturates in the control of symptoms in patients with terminal cancer. *Southern Medical Journal* 84:332–37.

Gregory, R. E., S. A. Grossman, V. R. Sheidler, and L. E. Wiggins. 1991. Seizures (SZ) associated with high-dose, intravenous (IV) morphine (MS) infusions: Incidence and possible etiology. *Proceedings of the American Society of Clinical Oncology* 10:335.

Groenewoud, J. H., A. van der Heide, B. D. Onwuteaka-Philipsen, D. L. Willems, P. J. van der Maas, and G. van der Wal. 2000. Clinical problems with the performance of euthanasia and physician-assisted suicide in the Netherlands. *New England Journal of Medicine* 342:551–56.

Haazen, L., H. Noorduin, A. Megens, and T. Meert. 1999. The constipation-inducing potential of morphine and transdermal fentanyl. *European Journal of Pain* 3(suppl. A):9–15.

Hanks, G. W. 1984. Psychotropic drugs. *Clinics in Oncology* 3:135–51.

Hanks, G. W. 1989. Controlled-release morphine (MST Contin) in advanced cancer: The European experience. *Cancer* 63:2378–82.

Hanks, G. W., and D. M. Justins. 1992. Cancer pain: Management. *Lancet* 339:1031–36.

Hanson, D., D. K. Langemo, B. Olson, S. Hunter, T. R. Sauvage, C. Burd, and T. Cathcart-Silberberg. 1991. The prevalence and incidence of pressure ulcers in the hospice setting: Analysis of two methodologies. *American Journal of Hospice and Palliative Care* 8:18–22.

Heilmann, K. 1978. Therapeutic systems for systemic use. In K. Heilmann, *Therapeutic Systems. Pattern-Specific Drug Delivery: Concept and Development,* 43–77. Stuttgart: Georg Thieme.

Henry, K., S. Rathgaber, C. Sullivan, and K. McCabe. 1992. Diabetes mellitus induced by megestrol acetate in a patient with AIDS and cachexia. *Annals of Internal Medicine* 116:53–54.

Herwig, K. R. 1980. Management of urinary incontinence and retention in the patient with advanced cancer. *Journal of the American Medical Association* 244:2203–4.

Higginson, I., and M. McCarthy. 1989. Measuring symptoms in terminal cancer: Are pain and dyspnea controlled? *Journal of the Royal Society of Medicine* 82:264–67.

Higginson, I., A. Wade, and M. McCarthy. 1990. Financial help for terminally ill patients. *Lancet* 1:172.

Hillner, B. E., J. N. Ingle, J. R. Berenson, N. A. Janjan, K. S. Albain, A. Lipton, G. Yee, J. S. Biermann, R. T. Chlebowski, and D. G. Pfister. 2000. American Society of Clinical Oncology guideline on the role of bisphosphonates in breast cancer. *Journal of Clinical Oncology* 18:1378–91.

Hockley, J. M., R. Dunlop, and R. J. Davies. 1988. Survey of distressing symptoms in dying patients and their families in hospital and the response to a symptom control team. *British Medical Journal* 296:1715–17.

Hoffman, M., A. Provatas, A. Lyver, and R. Kanner. 1991. Pain management in the opioid-addicted patient with cancer. *Cancer* 68:1121–22.

Hogan, C. M. 1986. Nausea and vomiting. In *Nursing Management of Symptoms Associated with Chemotherapy*, ed. J. M. Yasko, 57–71. Columbus, Ohio: Adria Laboratories.

Hogan, Q., D. E. Weissman, J. D. Haddox, S. Abram, M. L. Taylor, and N. Janjan. 1991. Epidural opiates and local anesthetics for the management of cancer pain. *Proceedings of the American Society of Clinical Oncology* 10:329.

Holland, J. C. 1987. Managing depression in the patient with cancer. *CA: A Cancer Journal for Clinicians* 37:366–71.

Holland, J. C., G. R. Morrow, A. Schmale, L. Derogatis, M. Stefanek, S. Berenson, P. J. Carpenter, W. Breitbart, and M. Feldstein. 1991. A randomized clinical trial of alprazolam versus progressive muscle relaxation in cancer patients with anxiety and depressive symptoms. *Journal of Clinical Oncology* 9:1004–11.

Holmes, V. F., F. Adams, and F. Fernandez. 1987. Respiratory dyskinesia due to antiemetic therapy in a cancer patient. *Cancer Treatment Reports* 71:415–16.

Hoskin, P. J., and G. W. Hanks. 1988. The management of symptoms in advanced cancer: Experience in a hospital-based continuing care unit. *Journal of the Royal Society of Medicine* 81:341–44.

Hoskin, P. J., and G. W. Hanks. 1990. Morphine: Pharmacokinetics and clinical practice. *British Journal of Cancer* 62:705–7.

Humphry, D. 1991. *Final Exit.* Eugene, Ore.: The Hemlock Society.

Husband, D. J. 1998. Malignant spinal cord compression: Prospective study of delays in referral and treatment. *British Medical Journal* 317:18–21.

Jacobsberg, L. B., and S. Perry. 1992. Psychiatric disturbances. *Medical Clinics of North America* 76:99–106.

Jacox, A., D. B. Carr, R. Payne, et al. 1994. *Management of Cancer Pain. Clinical Practice Guideline* No. 9. AHCPR Publication No. 94–0592. Rockville, Md.: Agency for Health Care Policy and Research, U. S. Department of Health and Human Services, Public Health Service.

Jaffe, J. H. 1985. Drug addiction and drug abuse. In *The Pharmacological Basis of*

Therapeutics, ed. A. G. Gilman, L. S. Goodman, T. W. Rall, and F. Murad, chapter 23. New York: Macmillan.

Jatoi, A., S. Kumar, J. A. Sloan, and P. L. Nguyen. 2000. On appetite and its loss. *Journal of Clinical Oncology* 18:2930–32.

Johanson, G. A. 1992. New routes of opioid administration. *American Journal of Hospice and Palliative Care* 9:4–5.

Joranson, D. E., K. M. Ryan, A. M. Gilson, and J. L. Dahl. 2000. Trends in medical use and abuse of opioid analgesics. *Journal of the American Medical Association* 282:1710–14.

Joshi, J. H., C. A. deJongh, N. Schnaper, C. L. Fortner, and P. H. Wiernik. 1982. Amphetamine therapy for enhancing the comfort of terminally ill patients (pts) with cancer. *Proceedings of the American Society of Clinical Oncology* 1:55.

Kaiko, R. F., S. L. Wallenstein, A. G. Rogers, P. Y. Grabinski, and R. W. Houde. 1982. Narcotics in the elderly. *Medical Clinics of North America* 66:1079–89.

Kaplan, L. D., C. B. Wofsy, and P. A. Volberding. 1987. Treatment of patients with acquired immunodeficiency syndrome and associated manifestations. *Journal of the American Medical Association* 257:1367–74.

Karnofsky, D. A., and J. H. Burchenal. 1949. The clinical evaluation of chemotherapeutic agents in cancer. In *Evaluation of Chemotherapeutic Agents,* ed. C. M. Macleod, 191–205. New York: Columbia University Press.

Kellar, M. 1984. A retrospective review of patients receiving continuous morphine infusion. *PRN Forum* 3:5–6.

Kerr, D. 1989. A bedside fan for terminal dyspnea. *American Journal of Hospice Care* 6:22.

Kerr, I. G., M. Sone, C. DeAngelis, N. Iscoe, R. MacKenzie, and T. Schueller. 1988. Continuous narcotic infusion with patient-controlled analgesia for chronic cancer pain in outpatients. *Annals of Internal Medicine* 108:554–57.

Kinzel, T. 1991. Managing lung disease in late life: A new approach. *Geriatrics* 46:54–59.

Krebs, H. B., and D. R. Goplerud. 1983. Surgical management of bowel obstruction in advanced ovarian carcinoma. *Obstetrics and Gynecology* 61:327–30.

Kris, M. G., S. D. J. Yeh, R. J. Gralla, and C. W. Young. 1985. Symptomatic gastroparesis in cancer patients: A possible cause of cancer-associated anorexia that can be improved with oral metoclopramide. *Proceedings of the American Society of Clinical Oncology* 4:267.

Lamer, T. J. 1994. Treatment of cancer-related pain: When orally administered medications fail. *Mayo Clinic Proceedings* 69:473–80.

Lamerton, R. 1991. Dehydration in dying patients. *Lancet* 337:981–82.

Langstein, H. N., and J. A. Norton. 1991. Mechanisms of cancer cachexia. *Hematology/Oncology Clinics of North America* 5:103–23.

Lawlor, P. G., B. Gagnon, I. L. Mancini, J. L. Pereira, J. Hanson, M. E. Suarez-Almazor, and E. Bruera. 2000. Occurrence, causes, and outcome of delirium in patients with advanced cancer. A prospective study. *Archives of Internal Medicine* 160:786–94.

Levick, S., C. Jacobs, D. F. Loukas, D. H. Gordon, F. L. Meyskens, and K. Uhm. 1988. Naproxen sodium in treatment of bone pain due to metastatic cancer. *Pain* 35:253–58.

Levine, P. M., P. M. Silberfarb, and Z. J. Lipowski. 1978. Mental disorders in cancer patients: A study of 100 psychiatric referrals. *Cancer* 42:1385–91.

Levy, D. E., J. J. Caronna, B. H. Singer, R. H. Lapinski, H. Frydman, and F. Plum. 1985. Predicting outcome from hypoxic-ischemic coma. *Journal of the American Medical Association* 253:1420–26.

Levy, M. H. 1996. Pharmacologic treatment of cancer pain. *New England Journal of Medicine* 335:1124–32.

Librach, S. L., and L. M. Rapson. 1988. The use of transcutaneous electrical nerve stimulation (TENS) for the relief of pain in palliative care. *Palliative Medicine* 2:15–20.

Lichter, I. 1990. Weakness in terminal illness. *Palliative Medicine* 4:73–80.

Lichter, I., and E. Hunt. 1990. The last 48 hours of life. *Journal of Palliative Care* 6:7–15.

Lindley, C. M., J. A. Dalton, and S. M. Fields. 1990. Narcotic analgesics: Clinical pharmacology and therapeutics. *Cancer Nursing* 13:28–38.

Lipman, A. G. 1989. Opioid analgesics in the management of cancer pain. *American Journal of Hospice Care* 6:13–23.

Lipman, A. G. 2000. New and alternative noninvasive opioid dosage forms and routes of administration. *Principles and Practice of Supportive Oncology Updates* 3:1–8.

Lipowski, Z. J. 1987. Delirium (acute confusional states). *Journal of the American Medical Association* 258:1789–92.

Lipowski, Z. J. 1989. Delirium in the elderly patient. *New England Journal of Medicine* 320:578–82.

Lo, B. 1991. Unanswered questions about DNR orders. *Journal of the American Medical Association* 265:1874–75.

Longstreth, W. T., T. S. Inui, L. A. Cobb, and M. K. Copass. 1983. Neurologic recovery after out-of-hospital cardiac arrest. *Annals of Internal Medicine* 98:588–92.

Loprinzi, C. L., N. M. Ellison, D. J. Schaid, J. E. Krook, L. M. Athmann, A. M. Dose, J. A. Mailliard, P. S. Johnson, L. P. Ebbert, and L. H. Geeraerts. 1990. Controlled trial of megestrol acetate for the treatment of cancer anorexia and cachexia. *Journal of National Cancer Institute* 82:1127–32.

Loprinzi, C. L., J. Mailliard, D. J. Schaid, J. E. Krook, R. M. Goldberg, M. Keppen, and J. Michalak. 1992. Dose/response evaluation of megestrol acetate (MA) for the treatment of cancer anorexia/cachexia: A Mayo Clinic and North Central Cancer Treatment Group Trial. *Proceedings of the American Society of Clinical Oncology* 11:378.

Loprinzi, C. L., J. W. Kugler, J. A. Sloan, J. A. Mailliard, J. E. Krook, M. B. Wilwerding, K. M. Rowland, J. K. Camoriano, P. J. Novotny, and B. J. Christensen. 1999. Randomized comparison of megestrol acetate versus dexamethasone versus fluoxymesterone for the treatment of cancer anorexia/cachexia. *Journal of Clinical Oncology* 17:3299–3306.

Lynn, J. 1986. Dying and dementia. *Journal of the American Medical Association* 256:2244–45.

Lynn, J. 1997. An 88-year-old woman facing the end of life. *Journal of the American Medical Association* 277:1633–40.

McCann, R. M., W. J. Hall, and A. Groth-Juncker. 1994. Comfort care for terminally ill patients: The appropriate use of hydration and nutrition. *Journal of the American Medical Association* 272:1263–66.

McNamara, P., M. Minton, and R. G. Twycross. 1991. Use of midazolam in palliative care. *Palliative Medicine* 5:244–49.

McQuay, H. 1998. Systematic reviews of pain therapies. In *2nd International Conference 1998—Comprehensive Cancer Care (ICCC)*, ed. S. Kaasa, 13–17. Limassol, Cyprus: Hadjigeorgiou Printing and Co., Ltd.

McQuay, H. 1999. Opioids in pain management. *Lancet* 353:2229–32.

McQuay, H., D. Carroll, A. R. Jadad, P. Wiffen, and A. Moore. 1995. Anticonvulsant drugs for management of pain: A systematic review. *British Medical Journal* 311:1047–52.

Magni, G., P. Conlon, and D. Arsie. 1987. Tricyclic antidepressants in the treatment of cancer pain: A review. *Pharmacopsychiatry* 20:160–64.

Maguire, L. C., J. L. Yon, and E. Miller. 1981. Prevention of narcotic induced constipation. *New England Journal of Medicine* 305:1651.

Maloney, C. M., R. K. Kesner, G. Klein, and J. Bockenstette. 1989. The rectal administration of MS Contin: Clinical implications of use in end stage cancer. *American Journal of Hospice Care* 6:34–35.

Mansour, R. P., H. A. Abdel-Rahman, and H. G. Wold. 1999. Retrospective review of slow release oral narcotic use in terminally ill cancer patients. *Proceedings of the American Society of Clinical Oncology* 18:583a.

Maouskop, A., N. Coyle, J. Maggard, and K. M. Foley. 1985. Continuous subcutaneous infusions of opiates in cancer patients with pain: Safety and efficacy. *Proceedings of the American Society of Clinical Oncology* 4:39.

Marin, J., M. C. Ilanez, and S. Arribas. 1990. Therapeutic management of nausea and vomiting. *General Pharmacology* 21:1–10.

Martin, D. K., L. L. Emanuel, and P. A. Singer. 2000. Planning for the end of life. *Lancet* 356:1672–76.

Massie, M. J., J. Holland, and E. Glass. 1983. Delirium in terminally ill cancer patients. *American Journal of Psychiatry* 140:1048–50.

Medical Letter. 1989a. Drugs that cause psychiatric symptoms. *Medical Letter* 31: 113–18.

Medical Letter. 1989b. Drugs for rheumatoid arthritis. *Medical Letter* 31:61–64.

Melzack, R., B. M. Mount, and J. M. Gordon. 1979. The Brompton mixture versus morphine solution given orally: Effects on pain. *Canadian Medical Association Journal* 120:435–38.

Miser, A. W., P. K. Narang, J. A. Dothage, R. C. Young, W. Sindelar, and J. S. Miser. 1989. Transdermal fentanyl for pain control in patients with cancer. *Pain* 37:15–21.

Mitsumoto, H., M. R. Hanson, and D. A. Chad. 1988. Amyotrophic lateral sclerosis: Recent advances in pathogenesis and therapeutic trials. *Archives of Neurology* 45:189–202.

Mocroft, A., M. Youle, J. Morcinek, C. A. Sabin, B. Gazzard, A. N. Phillips, and M. Johnson. 1997. Survival after diagnosis of AIDS: A prospective observational study of 2625 patients. *British Medical Journal* 314:409–20.

Moertel, C. G., A. J. Schutt, R. J. Reitemeier, and R. J. Hahn. 1974. Corticosteroid therapy of preterminal gastrointestinal cancer. *Cancer* 33:1607–9.

Morita, T., T. Ichiki, J. Tsunoda, S. Inoue, and S. Chihara. 1998. A prospective study on the dying process in terminally ill cancer patients. *American Journal of Hospice and Palliative Care* 15:217–22.

Morita, T., J. Tsunoda, S. Inoue, and S. Chihara. 2000. Terminal sedation for existential distress. *American Journal of Hospice and Palliative Care* 17:189–95.

Morris, J. N., S. Suissa, S. Sherwood, S. M. Wright, and D. Greer. 1986. Last days: A study of the quality of life of terminally ill cancer patients. *Journal of Chronic Disease* 39:47–62.

Morrison, R. S., and A. L. Siu. 2000. Survival in end-stage dementia following acute illness. *Journal of the American Medical Association* 284:47–52.

Moss, V. 1991. Patient characteristics, presentation, and problems encountered in advanced AIDS in a hospice setting: A review. *Palliative Medicine* 5:112–16.

Moulin, D. E., J. H. Kreeft, N. Murray-Parsons, and A. I. Bouquillon. 1991. Comparison of continuous subcutaneous and intravenous hydromorphone infusions for management of cancer pain. *Lancet* 337:465–68.

Muir, J. C. 1999. Malignant bowel obstruction. *Principles and Practice of Supportive Oncology Updates* 2:1–7.

Newman, V., M. Allwood, and R. A. Oakes. 1989. The use of metronidazole gel to control the smell of malodorous lesions. *Palliative Medicine* 3:303–5.

Nielsen, O. S., A. J. Munro, and I. F. Tannock. 1991. Bone metastases: Pathophysiology and management policy. *Journal of Clinical Oncology* 9:509–24.

O'Brien, T., M. Kelly, and C. Saunders. 1992. Motor neurone disease: A hospice perspective. *British Medical Journal* 304:471–73.

O'Brien, T., J. Welsh, and F. G. Dunn. 1998. Non-malignant conditions. *British Medical Journal* 316:286–89.

O'Neill, B., and M. Fallon. 1997. Principles of palliative care and pain control. *British Medical Journal* 315:801–4.

Osteen, R. T., S. Guyton, G. Steele, and R. E. Wilson. 1980. Malignant intestinal obstruction. *Surgery* 87:611–15.

Parkes, C. M. 2000. Commentary: Prognoses should be based on proved indices not intuition. *British Medical Journal* 320:473.

Pass, H. I., and J. A. Roth. 1987. Diagnosis of pulmonary metastases. In *Surgical Treatment of Metastatic Disease,* ed. S. A. Rosenberg, chapter 2. Philadelphia: J. B. Lippincott.

Payne, R. 1987a. Novel routes of opioid administration in the management of cancer pain. *Oncology* 1:10–18.

Payne, R. 1987b. Role of epidural and intrathecal narcotics and peptides in the management of cancer pain. *Medical Clinics of North America* 71:313–27.

Payne, R. 1989a. Novel routes of opioid administration, part 5: Spinal epidural and intrathecal. *Primary Care and Cancer* 9:31–32.

Payne, R. 1989b. Pharmacologic management of bone pain in the cancer patient. *Clinical Journal of Pain* 5(Suppl. 2):S43–50.

Payne, R. 1991. Pain. In *Manual of Oncologic Therapeutics, 1991/1992,* ed. R. E. Wittes, chapter 57. Philadelphia: J. B. Lippincott.

Payne, R. 1992. Transdermal fentanyl: Suggested recommendations for clinical use. *Journal of Pain and Symptom Management* 7:540–44.

Payne, R. 1999. Titrating opioids and converting to long-acting agents. *Oncology* 13:581–86.

Payne, R., S. D. Mathias, D. J. Pasta, L. A. Wanke, R. Williams, and R. Mahmoud. 1998. Quality of life and cancer pain: Satisfaction and side effects with transdermal fentanyl versus oral morphine. *Journal of Clinical Oncology* 16:1588–93.

Penn, R. D., and J. A. Paice. 1987. Chronic intrathecal morphine for intractable pain. *Journal of Neurosurgery* 67:182–86.

Peteet, J., V. Tay, G. Cohen, and J. MacIntyre. 1986. Pain characteristics and treatment in an outpatient cancer population. *Cancer* 57:1259–65.

Peters, R. C. D. U. 1997. Neuroaugmentative procedures for pain. Personal Communication.

Phillips, H. 1984. Orthopaedic surgery. *Clinics in Oncology* 3:75–87.

Phillips, L. L. 1998. Managing the pain of bone metastases in the home environment. *American Journal of Hospice and Palliative Care* 15:32–42.

Pirl, W. F., and A. J. Roth. 1999. Diagnosis and treatment of depression in cancer patients. *Oncology* 13:1293–1301.

Pitorak, E. F., and J. C. Kraus. 1987. Pain control with sublingual morphine: The advantages for hospice care. *American Journal of Hospice Care* 4:39–41.

Plezia, P. M., T. H. Kramer, J. Linford, and S. R. Hameroff. 1989. Transdermal fentanyl: Pharmacokinetics and preliminary clinical evaluation. *Pharmacotherapy* 9:2–9.

Popiela, T., R. Lucchi, and F. Giongo. 1989. Methylprednisolone as palliative therapy for female terminal cancer patients. *European Journal of Cancer and Clinical Oncology* 25:1823–29.

Portenoy, R. K. 1987. Constipation in the cancer patient: Causes and management. *Medical Clinics of North America* 71:303–11.

Portenoy, R. K. 1990. Drug therapy for cancer pain. *American Journal of Hospice and Palliative Care* 7:10–19.

Portenoy, R. K. 1998. Principles of opioid pharmacotherapy and Nonopioids and adjuvant analgesics. In R. K. Portenoy, *Pain in Oncologic and AIDS Patients*, chapters 4 and 6. Newtown: Handbooks in Healthcare Co.

Portenoy, R. K., and P. Lesage. 1999. Management of cancer pain. *Lancet* 353:1695–1700.

Portenoy, R. K., D. E. Moulin, A. Rogers, C. E. Inturrisi, and K. M. Foley. 1986. IV infusion of opioids for cancer pain: Clinical review and guidelines for use. *Cancer Treatment Reports* 70:575–81.

Posner, J. B. 1979. Neurological complications of systemic cancer. *Medical Clinics of North America* 63:783–800.

Potter, W. Z., M. V. Rudorfer, and H. Manji. 1991. The pharmacologic treatment of depression. *New England Journal of Medicine* 325:633–42.

Poulsen, H. S., O. S. Nielsen, M. Klee, and M. Rorth. 1989. Palliative irradiation of bone metastases. *Cancer Treatment Reviews* 16:41–48.

Powell, N. 1979. Tao: The Chinese way. In N. Powell, *The Book of Change: How to Understand and Use the I. Ching*, chapter 1. London: Macdonald and Company.

President's Commission for the Study of Ethical Problems in Medicine and Biomedical and Behavioral Research. 1983. *Deciding to forego life-sustaining treat-*

ment: A report on the ethical, medical, and legal issues in treatment decisions. Washington, D. C.: U. S. Government Printing Office.

Quill, T. E. 1991. Death and dignity: A case of individualized decision making. *New England Journal of Medicine* 324:691–94.

Quill, T. E., and I. R. Byock. 2000. Responding to intractable terminal suffering: The role of terminal sedation and voluntary refusal of food and fluids. *Annals of Internal Medicine* 132:408–14.

Quill, T. E., B. C. Lee, and S. Nunn. 2000. Palliative treatments of last resort: Choosing the least harmful alternative. *Annals of Internal Medicine* 132:488–93.

Ray, W. A., M. R. Griffin, W. Schaffner, D. K. Baugh, and L. J. Melton. 1987. Psychotropic drug use and the risk of hip fracture. *New England Journal of Medicine* 316:363–69.

Redfield, R. R., and E. C. Tramont. 1989. Toward a better classification system for HIV infection. *New England Journal of Medicine* 320:1414–16.

Rees, W. D., S. B. Dover, and T. S. Low-Beer. 1987. "Patients with terminal cancer" who have neither terminal illness nor cancer. *British Medical Journal* 295:318–19.

Regnard, C. 1988. The treatment of bowel obstruction in advanced cancer: An algorithm. *Palliative Medicine* 2:131–33.

Regnard, C., and S. Ahmedzai. 1991. Dyspnoea in advanced nonmalignant disease: A flow diagram. *Palliative Medicine* 5:56–60.

Regnard, C., and K. Mannix. 1991. Urinary problems in advanced cancer: A flow diagram. *Palliative Medicine* 5:344–48.

Rcitmeier, M., and R. C. Hartenstein. 1990. Megestrolacetate and determination of body composition by bioelectrical impedance analysis in cancer cachexia. *Proceedings of the American Society of Clinical Oncology* 9:325.

Reuben, D. B., and V. Mor. 1986a. Dyspnea in terminally ill cancer patients. *Chest* 89:234–36.

Reuben, D. B., and V. Mor. 1986b. Nausea and vomiting in terminal cancer patients. *Archives of Internal Medicine* 146:2021–23.

Reuben, D. B., V. Mor, and J. Hiris. 1988. Clinical symptoms and length of survival in patients with terminal cancer. *Archives of Internal Medicine* 148:1586–91.

Reuler, J. B., and T. G. Cooney. 1981. The pressure sore: Pathophysiology and principles of management. *Annals of Internal Medicine* 94:661–66.

Rhymes, J. A., L. B. McCullough, R. J. Luchi, T. A. Teasdale, and N. Wilson. 2000. Withdrawing very low-burden interventions in chronically ill patients. *Journal of the American Medical Association* 283:1061–63.

Richardson, M. A., T. Sanders, J. L. Palmer, A. Greisinger, and S. E. Singletary. 2000. Complementary/alternative medicine use in a comprehensive cancer center and implications for oncology. *Journal of Clinical Oncology* 18:2505–14.

Riesenberg, D. 2000. Hospital care of patients with dementia. *Journal of the American Medical Association* 284:87–89.

Ripamonti, C. 1998. Patient-controlled analgesia in cancer pain. In *2nd International Conference 1998—Comprehensive Cancer Care (ICCC)*, ed. S. Kaasa, 23–25. Limassol, Cyprus: Hadjigeorgiou Printing and Co., Ltd.

Ripamonti, C., L. Groff, C. Brunelli, D. Polastri, A. Stavrakis, and F. De Conno.

1998. Switching from morphine to oral methadone in treating cancer pain: What is the equianalgesic dose ratio? *Journal of Clinical Oncology* 16: 3216–21.

Ripamonti, C., A. Filiberti, A. Totis, F. De Conno, and M. Tamburini. 1999. Suicide among patients with cancer cared for at home by palliative-care teams. *Lancet* 354:1877–78.

Rivlin, R. S., M. E. Shils, and P. Sherlock. 1983. Nutrition and cancer. *American Journal of Medicine* 75:843–54.

Rowbotham, M., N. Harden, B. Stacey, P. Bernstein, and L. Magnus-Miller. 1998. Gabapentin for the treatment of postherpetic neuralgia. A randomized controlled trial. *Journal of the American Medical Association* 280:1837–42.

Rowland, C. G., and K. M. Pagliero. 1985. Intracavitary irradiation in palliation of carcinoma of oesophagus and cardia. *Lancet* 2:981–83.

Rowlingson, J. C., R. J. Hamill, and R. B. Patt. 1993. Comprehensive assessment of the patient with cancer pain. In *Cancer Pain,* ed. R. B. Patt, chapter 2. Philadelphia: J. B. Lippincott.

Roy, D. J. 1990. Need they sleep before they die? *Journal of Palliative Care* 6:3–4.

Ryan, T. J. 1989. Pressure sores: Prevention, management and future research— a medical perspective. *Palliative Medicine* 3:249–55.

Sallerin-Caute, B., Y. Lazorthes, O. Deguine, B. Frances, J.-C. Verdie, J.-P. Charlet, and R. Bastide. 1998. Does intrathecal morphine in the treatment of cancer pain induce the development of tolerance? *Neurosurgery* 42:44–50.

Sandgren, J. E., M. S. McPhee, and N. J. Greenberger. 1984. Narcotic bowel syndrome treated with clonidine: Resolution of abdominal pain and intestinal pseudo-obstruction. *Annals of Internal Medicine* 101:331–34.

Saunders, C. 1982. Principles of symptom control in terminal care. *Medical Clinics of North America* 66:1169–83.

Saunders, C. 1984. Pain and impending death. In *Textbook of Pain,* ed. P. D. Wall and R. Melzack, 472–78. Edinburgh: Churchill Livingstone.

Saunders, C., T. D. Walsh, and M. Smith. 1981. Hospice care in motor neuron disease. In *Hospice: The Living Idea,* ed. C. Saunders, D. H. Summers, and N. Teller, chapter 6. London: Edward Arnold.

Sawe, J., B. Dahlstrom, L. Paalzow, and A. Rane. 1981. Morphine kinetics in cancer patients. *Clinical Pharmacology and Therapeutics* 30:629–35.

Schell, H. W. 1972. Adrenal corticosteroid therapy in far-advanced cancer. *Geriatrics* 27:131–41.

Schonwetter, R., and C. R. Jani. 2000. Survival estimation in noncancer patients with advanced disease. In *Topics in Palliative Care,* ed. R. K. Portenoy and E. Bruera, chapter 3. New York: Oxford University Press.

Seamans, D. P., G. Y. Wong, and J. L. Wilson. 2000. Interventional pain therapy for intractable abdominal cancer pain. *Journal of Clinical Oncology* 18:1598–1600.

Seigel, L. J., and D. L. Longo. 1981. The control of chemotherapy-induced emesis. *Annals of Internal Medicine* 95:352–59.

Sharp, K. W., and E. J. Stevens. 1991. Improving palliation in pancreatic cancer: Intraoperative celiac plexus block for pain relief. *Southern Medical Journal* 84:469–71.

Silverstein, M. D., C. B. Stocking, J. P. Antel, J. Beckwith, R. P. Roos, and M. Seigler. 1991. Amyotrophic lateral sclerosis and life-sustaining therapy: Patients' desires for information, participation in decision making and life-sustaining therapy. *Mayo Clinic Proceedings* 66:906–13.

Simmonds, M. A., R. Payne, J. Richenbacher, K. Moran, and M. A. Southam. 1989. TTS (fentanyl) in the management of pain in patients with cancer. *Proceedings of the American Society of Clinical Oncology* 8:324.

Smith, T. J., and K. Swisher. 1998. Telling the truth about terminal cancer. *Journal of the American Medical Association* 279:1746–48.

Socher, S. H., D. Martinez, J. B. Craig, J. G. Kuhn, and A. Oliff. 1988. Tumor necrosis factor not detectable in patients with clinical cancer cachexia. *Journal of the National Cancer Institute* 80:595–98.

Sorensen, P. S., S. E. Borgesen, K. Rohde, B. Rasmusson, F. Bach, T. Boge-Rasmussen, P. Stjernholm, B. H. Larson, N. Agerlin, and F. Gjerris. 1990. Metastatic epidural spinal cord compression: Results of treatment and survival. *Cancer* 65:1502–8.

Stedeford, A., and C. Regnard. 1991. Confusional states in advanced cancer: A flow diagram. *Palliative Medicine* 5:256–61.

Steiner, I., and T. Siegal. 1989. Muscle cramps in cancer patients. *Cancer* 63:574–77.

Steitz, A. M. 1987. Analgesic utilization patterns in a hospice. *Oncology* 1:33–36.

Stone, T. H., and W. J. Winslade. 1995. Physician-assisted suicide and euthanasia in the United States. *Journal of Legal Medicine* 16:481–507.

Streisand, J. B., J. R. Varvel, D. R. Stanski, L. L. Marie, M. A. Ashburn, B. I. Hague, S. D. Tarver, and T. H. Stanley. 1991. Absorption and bioavailability of oral transmucosal fentanyl citrate. *Anesthesiology* 75:223–29.

Sugibayashi, K., C. Sakanoue, and Y. Morimoto. 1989. Utility of topical formulations of morphine hydrochloride containing azone and N-methyl-2-pyrrolidone. *Selective Cancer Therapeutics* 5:119–28.

Sullivan, A. D., K. Hedberg, and D. W. Fleming. 2000. Legalized physician-assisted suicide in Oregon—The second year. *New England Journal of Medicine* 342:598–604.

Sundaresan, N., G. V. DiGiacinto, and J. E. O. Hughes. 1989. Neurosurgery in the treatment of cancer pain. *Cancer* 63:2365–77.

SUPPORT Principal Investigators. 1995. A controlled trial to improve care for seriously ill hospitalized patients: The Study to Understand Prognoses and Preferences for Outcomes and Risks of Treatments (SUPPORT). *Journal of the American Medical Association* 274:1591–98.

Swanson, G., J. Smith, R. Bulich, P. New, and R. Shiffman. 1989. Patient-controlled analgesia for chronic cancer pain in the ambulatory setting: A report of 117 patients. *Journal of Clinical Oncology* 7:1903–8.

Sykes, J., R. Johnson, and G. W. Hanks. 1997. Difficult pain problems. *British Medical Journal* 315:867–69.

Sykes, N. P. 1991. A clinical comparison of laxatives in a hospice. *Palliative Medicine* 5:307–14.

Sykes, N. P., R. L. Carter, and M. Baines. 1988. Clinical and pathological study of dysphagia conservatively managed in patients with advanced malignant disease. *Lancet* 2:726–28.

Tannock, I., M. Gospodarowicz, W. Meakin, T. Panzarella, L. Stewart, and W. Rider. 1989. Treatment of metastatic prostatic cancer with low-dose prednisone: Evaluation of pain and quality of life as pragmatic indices of response. *Journal of Clinical Oncology* 7:590–97.

Tchekmedyian, N. S., N. Tait, M. Moody, and J. Aisner. 1987. High-dose megestrol acetate: A possible treatment for cachexia. *Journal of the American Medical Association* 257:1195–98.

Temple, W. J., and A. S. Ketcham. 1990. Surgical palliation for recurrent rectal cancers ulcerating in the perineum. *Cancer* 65:1111–14.

Thirlwell, M. P., P. A. Sloan, J. A. Maroun, G. J. Boors, J. G. Besner, J. H. Stewart, and B. M. Mount. 1989. Pharmacokinetics and clinical efficacy of oral morphine solution and controlled-release morphine tablets in cancer patients. *Cancer* 63:2275–83.

Thorns, A., and N. Sykes. 2000. Opioid use in last week of life and implications for end-of-life decision-making. *Lancet* 356:398–99.

Toscani, F., K. Barosi, S. Camerini and M. Gallucci. 1989. Sodium naproxen: Continuous subcutaneous infusion in neoplastic pain control. *Palliative Medicine* 3:207–11.

Turnbull, A. D. M., J. Guerra, and H. F. Starnes. 1989. Results of surgery for obstructing carcinomatosis of gastrointestinal, pancreatic or biliary origin. *Journal of Clinical Oncology* 7:381–86.

Twycross, R. G., and G. W. Hanks. 1984. Co-analgesia. *Clinics in Oncology* 3:153–64.

U. S. General Accounting Office. 1989. Hospice participation in Medicare: Executive summary. In GAO/HRD-89-111. In *Hospice Participation in Medicare,* 2–5. Washington D. C.: Government Printing Office.

Vainio, A., J. Ollila, E. Matikainen, P. Rosenberg, and E. Kalso. 1995. Driving ability in cancer patients receiving long-term morphine analgesia. *Lancet* 346:667–70.

Van Dam, J., and W. R. Brugge. 1999. Endoscopy of the upper gastrointestinal tract. *New England Journal of Medicine* 341:1738–48.

Van Holten-Verzantvoort, A. T., O. L. M. Bijvoet, J. Hermans, H. I. J. Harinck, J. W. F. Elte, L. V. A. M. Beex, F. J. Cleton, H. M. Kroon, P. Vermey, J. P. Neist, and G. Blijham. 1987. Reduced morbidity from skeletal metastases in breast cancer patients during long-term bisphosphonate (APD) treatment. *Lancet* 2:983–85.

Veith, I. 1972. *The Yellow Emperor's Classic of Internal Medicine.* Berkeley: University of California Press.

Ventafridda, V., M. Tamburini, A. Caraceni, F. De Conno, and F. Naldi. 1987. A validation study of the WHO method for cancer pain relief. *Cancer* 59:850–56.

Ventafridda, V., C. Ripamonti, A. Caraceni, E. Spoldi, L. Messina, and F. De Conno. 1990a. The management of inoperable gastrointestinal obstruction in terminal cancer patients. *Tumori* 76:389–93.

Ventafridda, V., C. Ripamonti, F. De Conno, M. Tamburini, and B. R. Cassileth. 1990b. Symptom prevalence and control during cancer patients' last days of life. *Journal of Palliative Care* 6:7–11.

Veronesi, V. 1982. Noncurative surgery. In *Cancer Medicine,* ed. J. F. Holland and E. Frei, section IX-4. Philadelphia: Lea & Febiger.

Vohra, R. K., and C. N. McCollum. 1994. Pressure sores. *British Medical Journal* 309:853–57.

Volicer, L., Y. Rheaume, J. Brown, K. Fabiszewski, and R. Brady. 1986. Hospice approach to the treatment of patients with advanced dementia of the Alzheimer type. *Journal of the American Medical Association* 256:2210–13.

Von Roenn, J. H., R. L. Murphy, and N. Wegener. 1990. Megestrol acetate for treatment of anorexia and cachexia associated with human immunodeficiency virus infection. *Seminars in Oncology* 6(supp. 9):13–16.

Von Roenn, J. H., R. L. Murphy, K. M. Weber, L. M. Williams, and S. A. Weitzman. 1988. Megestrol acetate for treatment of cachexia associated with human immunodeficiency virus (HIV) infection. *Annals of Internal Medicine* 109:840–41.

Wadleigh, R., M. Spaulding, B. Lembersky, M. Zimmer, K. Shepard, and T. Plasse. 1990. Dronabinol enhancement of appetite in cancer patients. *Proceedings of the American Society of Clinical Oncology* 9:331.

Waller, A., A. Adunski, and M. Hershkowitz. 1991. Terminal dehydration and intravenous fluids. *Lancet* 337:745.

Walsh, D. 1993. Dyspnoea in advanced cancer. *Lancet* 342:450–51.

Walsh, J. S., G. Welch, and E. B. Larson. 1990. Survival of outpatients with Alzheimer-type dementia. *Annals of Internal Medicine* 113:429–34.

Warrington, P. S., S. G. Allan, M. A. Cornbleet, J. S. MacPherson, J. F. Smyth, and R. C. F. Leonard. 1986. Optimizing antiemesis in cancer chemotherapy: Efficacy of continuous versus intermittent infusion of high dose metoclopramide in emesis induced by cisplatin. *British Medical Journal* 293:1334–37.

Watson, C. P., R. J. Evans, K. Reed, H. Merskey, L. Goldsmith, and J. Warsh. 1982. Amitriptyline versus placebo in postherpetic neuralgia. *Neurology* 32:671–73.

Weeks, J. C., E. F. Cook, S. J. O'Day, L. M. Peterson, N. Wenger, D. Reding, F. E. Harrell, P. Kussin, N. V. Dawson, A. F. Connors, J. Lynn, and R. S. Phillips. 1998. Relationship between cancer patients' predictions of prognosis and their treatment preferences. *Journal of the American Medical Association* 279:1709–14.

Weiss, S. H. 1992. HIV infection and the healthcare worker. *Medical Clinics of North America* 76:269–280.

Weissman, D. E., J. L. Dahl, and D. E. Joranson. 1990. Oral morphine for the treatment of cancer pain. *Principles and Practice of Oncology Updates* 6:1–8.

Weissman, D. E, D. E. Joranson, and M. Hopwood. 1991. The influence of drug regulations on opioid analgesic prescribing practice. *Proceedings of the American Society of Clinical Oncology* 10:321.

Wells, J. C. D. 1989. The use of nerve destruction for relief of pain in cancer: A review. *Palliative Medicine* 3:239–47.

White, I. D., P. J. Hoskins, G. W. Hanks, and J. M. Bliss. 1989. Morphine and dryness of the mouth. *British Medical Journal* 298:1222–23.

White, I. D., P. J. Hoskins, G. W. Hanks, and J. M. Bliss. 1991. Analysis in cancer pain: Current practice and beliefs. *British Journal of Cancer* 63:271–74.

White, P. F. 1988. Use of patient-controlled analgesia for management of acute pain. *Journal of the American Medical Association* 259:243–47.

Wilkes, E. 1974. Some problems in cancer management. *Proceedings of the Royal Society of Medicine* 67:1001–5.

Williams, D. B., and A. J. Windebank. 1991. Motor neuron disease (amyotrophic lateral sclerosis). *Mayo Clinic Proceedings* 66:54–82.

Willox, J. C., J. Corr, J. Shaw, M. Richardson, K. C. Calman, and M. Drennan. 1984. Prednisolone as an appetite stimulant in patients with cancer. *British Medical Journal* 288:27.

Wolf, S. M., P. Boyle, D. Callahan, J. J. Fins, B. Jennings, J. L. Nelson, J. A. Barondess, D. W. Brock, R. Dresser, L. Emanuel, S. Johnson, J. Lantos, D. R. Mason, M. Mezey, D. Orentlicher, and F. Rouse. 1991. Sources of concern about the Patient Self-Determination Act. *New England Journal of Medicine* 325:1666–71.

Wolfe, M. M., D. R. Lichenstein, and G. Singh. 1999. Gastrointestinal toxicity of nonsteroidal antiinflammatory drugs. *New England Journal of Medicine* 340:1888–99.

Wood, C. G. A., S. Whittet, and C. S. Bradbeer. 1997. HIV infection and AIDS. *British Medical Journal* 315:1433–36.

Wood, D. K. 1980. The draining malignant ulceration: Palliative management in advanced cancer. *Journal of the American Medical Association* 244:820–22.

Woodruff, R. 1997. Genitourinary. In R. Woodruff, *Symptom Control in Advanced Cancer,* chapter 4. Melbourne: Asperula Pty, Ltd.

Wrenn, K. 1989. Fecal impaction. *New England Journal of Medicine* 321:658–62.

Yarchoan, R., and S. Broder. 1987. Development of antiretroviral therapy for the acquired immunodeficiency syndrome and related disorders. *New England Journal of Medicine* 316:557–64.

Yates, J. W., B. Chalmer, and F. P. McKegney. 1980. Evaluation of patients with advanced cancer using the Karnofsky performance status. *Cancer* 45:2220–24.

Yuan, C. -S., J. F. Foss, M. O'Connor, J. Osinski, T. Karrison, J. Moss, and M. F. Roizen. 2000. Methylnaltrexone for reversal of constipation due to chronic methadone use. A randomized clinical trial. *Journal of the American Medical Association* 283:367–72.

Zerwekh, J. V. 1987. Should fluid and nutritional support be withheld from terminally ill patients?: Another opinion. *American Journal of Hospice Care* 4:37–38.

Index

Page numbers in *italics* denote figures; those followed by "t" denote tables.